Inner Ear Balance and Dizziness Disorders

To order additional copies, please contact us.
BookSurge, LLC
www.booksurge.com
1-866-308-6235
orders@booksurge.com

Inner Ear Balance and Dizziness Disorders

P.J. Haybach

2005

Inner Ear Balance and Dizziness Disorders

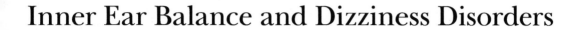

TABLE OF CONTENTS

To My Parents Who Always Stood By Me

Chapter One
Introduction

If you're reading these words chances are you're dizzy or have a balance problem going on and lots of questions are racing through your mind.

- What are all these sensations?
- Where is this coming from?
- What do I have?
- Who should I go to?
- What can be done?
- Why can't they just cut something out?
- When will it stop?
- Will I get well?

There just aren't any quick, easy answers to these questions, I'm afraid, but this book should help you begin to navigate through the minefield you may be lost in. I'll explain the mysteries of the ear and it's role in balance, things that can go wrong with the ear, what can be done about them and how to live with the changes. There really are things that can be tried no matter what you've been told. Even when there is no cure available there are ways to get some improvement or degree of relief, *in most cases.*

Luckily an inner ear balance problem is only a temporary blip on life's radar screen that quickly fades to nothing more than a bad memory, *for most people.* If your symptoms have just begun you most likely will recover quickly and won't ever look at this book again.

If you are one of the unfortunate people with a more lingering problem I'm sorry you need this book but it's written with you in mind and is bound to have something you'll find helpful.

> **Caution:** If you don't have a doctor or other health care provider, get one. Don't try to replace them with this book.

For those of you with normal ears this book can give a small look at the disorienting and frightening world of imbalance and dizziness, but only a peak. To really "get it" an inner ear balance disorder has got to be lived and felt minute-to-minute, hour-to-hour, day-to-day for weeks to years on end. Simply reading about it loses a little something in the translation, but it's better than nothing.

Organization of the book

This book contains both general and specific information about vestibular disorders. The first few chapters provide information about the health care system and the inner ear followed by diagnosis and treatment chapters and then specific vestibular disorders are described. More general information about the affects of vestibular disorders and how to deal with them follow in the last few chapters.

A word about dizziness

Unfortunately the words dizzy and dizziness don't have an exact meaning in the real or health care worlds. They seem to include any or all of a number of weird sensations; lightheadedness, faintness, movement illusions, feelings of non-reality, floating, swimming, or rocking sensations, spinning, nausea and queasiness, to name a few.

Dizziness is only in the title of this book because it's used by so many people to describe the abnormal sensations that go along with inner ear balance disorders. It's not used because it's a diagnosis or has a specific meaning.

When describing how you feel, particularly to a health care professional, stay away from a term like "dizzy" and say exactly what you are feeling. If you're feeling lightheaded and nauseated, say it. If you feel like you're spinning, say that. Always be as specific as possible, don't make the mistake of assuming people understand what you're talking about, there's a good chance they don't but are just nodding their heads because they were taught to be reassuring.

Chapter Two
Whom Should I Go To?

"Whom should I go to?" Great question—complicated answer. Finding the right doctor is tough and in the end may require more luck than anything else but reading through this chapter might just improve your chances.

The Players
Primary Care Provider (PCP)
This health care professional looks at a person as someone with a mind, soul and complete set of interacting body parts. They can be a medical doctor (MD), osteopathic doctor (OD), adult or family nurse practitioner (ANP or FNP) or physician's assistant (PA). They may treat you on their own or along with a specialist.

Specialists
Medical care is organized around the various areas and systems of the human body. A primary care provider is more or less responsible for the entire body. For the more complicated problems the body is then divided up amongst the various specialists. The ear happens to fall within the area of otolaryngology-head and neck surgery. Yes, surgery. We'll get into that a bit more in a minute.

Otolaryngologists (ENT's)
Otolaryngologists, many times referred to as ENT's (ear, nose and throat) since it's much easier to say, deal with everything above the shoulders except the brain, mind, eyes and teeth. This is a huge amount of territory with lots of disorders. Cancer of the mouth, tongue, throat and voice box; plastic surgery for cleft lip and palate; nosebleeds and broken noses; tonsils, sinuses, sometimes allergy work, facial bone fractures, thyroid removal, broken jaws, salivary gland problems, external ear infections, difficulty swallowing, taste disturbances, difficulty with speech, some esophagus problems, middle ear infections, eustachian tube dysfunction, ear balance and hearing problems, and even more, are all included in this specialty.

Doctors become board certified in otolaryngology-head and neck surgery after completing a long residency program and successfully passing both written and oral tests. They can then place the initials FACS after their name (fellow in the American College of Surgery) and may be referred to as a Diplomate of the American College of Surgery. These residency programs are regulated by the American Board of Medical Specialties, ABMS. They can't even enter the residency until completing their basic medical education that includes four years of college, four years of medical school and one year of a general internship throughout a hospital.

The first step in becoming an otolaryngologist after the internship is a one-year general surgery residency. This is followed by four years in an otolaryngology residency.

A residency program is really an on-the-job training course or apprenticeship for doctors. They are on duty long hours each week; we're talking around 80, and learn by working under other residents a year or two their senior and under experienced doctors who have previously completed a residency program.

Most of their time in training is spent hunched over the operating table learning and practicing all the skills needed to be a competent surgeon. The remaining time is used to learn about the diagnosis and non-surgical treatment of all the ear, nose, throat, head and neck disorders.

Despite all this, some otolaryngologists do good work with ear balance disorders. Others just don't have the education or experience to be effective, particularly in complicated cases or when symptoms don't fit the "textbook" description. Because the structure and function of the ear are so specialized and complicated there are sub-specialties within otolaryngology-head and neck surgery that focus just on the ear and the inner ear.

Otologists and Neurotologists

There are two sub-specialties for the ear, otology and neurotology. Otology covers all aspects of the ear and neurotology covers the inner ear and its role in balance and hearing. Although in theory these are different areas of expertise, in practice most ear doctors are both otologists and neurotologists.

> **Note:** Anyone can call himself or herself an otologist or neurotologist because the government doesn't regulate the use of the titles.

Many doctors using the title have undergone further training, beyond their residency, called a fellowship. A fellowship is another formal on-the-job program that takes place after a residency and board certification are completed. During fellowship training a doctor spends their time learning about the ear and it's disorders along with diagnosis and treatment from an experienced otologist/neurotologist and they also learn by doing. This training lasts one to two years and again generally includes a lot of time learning surgery.

These fellowships were not standardized nor was certification testing offered until the American Board of Otolaryngology (www.aboto.org) began testing in 2004. Very few doctors have been certified through this new process.

Different fellowship programs have different focuses with some preparing doctors to do scientific research or teach in a university and others focusing more on skills for private practice.

Not everyone who has successfully completed a fellowship in otology or neurotology limits his or her practice to these areas. Many continue to practice in other areas of the otolaryngology-head and neck specialty. To make sure a doctor only practices on folks with ear disorders ask if they **limit** their practice to ear disorders, not if they specialize in them.

> **In depth:** Otolaryngology-head and neck surgery is a specialty, doctors practicing it are specialists and anything within their specialty is what they specialize in. If you ask, "Do you specialize in inner ear balance disorders?" the answer of yes from anyone board certified as an otolaryngologist is honest even if it is only one of many areas they practice in.

Other Specialties
Neurologists can medically treat balance disorders caused by the brain or nervous system and neurosurgeons can treat them surgically.

A handful of neurologists limit their practice to people with ear balance problems, trouble arising in the nerves sending the balance information to the brain or a problem in the area of the brain receiving the balance information. Many times they are referred to as otoneurologists.

So, Whom Should I Go To?
First Stop
A primary care provider whom knows you well is a good first stop. They can check you out and if unable to help can recommend someone who might. Later on they can also help carry out medical therapies suggested by a specialist.

Sounds easy enough, right? Wrong. One problem here is that ear balance disorders are such a specialized little area of medicine some primary care providers don't even know enough about it to select the best specialist. An MD's basic education just doesn't have much in it about the ear or it's balance disorders. Most medical schools only require an hour or two of general lectures about the ear in their entire 4-year curriculum.

Another sticky little problem is that most doctors will refer their patients to other doctors in their group or medical building or at the hospital they practice in and not necessarily to the best guy available in the area. If you want to see the very best, ask for it.

Of course the ever-present insurance menace can also rear its ugly head here. An HMO (Health Maintenance Organization) or PPO (Preferred provider organization) insurance company will start you off by seeing one of their primary care providers. Then, if they determine a specialist is needed it will be with whomever they have a contract. Sometimes this happens to be the best person in the area; other times it's someone without special training or experience in inner ear balance disorders who might even dislike seeing "dizzy" people.

If this happens to you don't take it lying down. Complain in writing and by phone. Tell the insurance people who the proper specialist is. Not good at insisting? Don't be bashful; enlist the help of a relative or friend who's good at it.

Second Stop: The Specialist
So you or your primary care provider have determined a specialist is needed—which type and whom? There's a lot to consider here.

- Will you rely on advice and information from a health care professional, other people with the same problem or will you go it alone?
- Which type of specialist?
- What's available in your neck of the woods?
- Will your insurance pay or decide?

The easiest thing to do is have a primary care provider decide whom you should go to. Relying on their experience will lift a burden from your shoulders and leave less to worry about.

Don't want to leave this in the hands of someone else? That's OK but you'll have to accept a bit more work and soul searching. You can go it totally alone or hook up with other people having similar problems.

Finding people with similar problems can be done via the Internet or by joining the Vestibular Disorders Association (VEDA) for a small fee. They'll send out their "Link Lists" with the names of folks with ear balance problems willing to be contacted. In addition they also have lists of local support groups. The addresses for VEDA are PO Box 13305, Portland, OR 97213-0305,

Phone (24-hour voice mail): (800) 837-8428 and (503) 229-7705, Fax: (503) 229-8064 and www. vestibular.org, memberinfo@vestibular.org

There are several organized groups of people with ear balance problems on the Internet. Their addresses can change quite frequently and aren't listed here but you can find them listed at the VEDA web page.

The Meniere's Network at the Ear Foundation can also supply names of Meniere's support groups and other services. Their addresses are www.theearfound.com, PO Box 330867, Nashville, TN 37203, Phone Toll Free (voice/TDD): 1-800-545-HEAR, Phone (voice/TDD): 615-627-2724, Fax: 615-627-2728, and info@earfoundation.org

Contact some of the members of these organizations in your area and find out what they have to say about doctors they've been to. Who better to speak to than people who have been there, done that?

If you decide to go it alone you'll need to find an otologist, neurotologist or board certified general otolaryngologist. But whom?

The yellow pages will list otolaryngologists and otologists in their "Physician's and Surgeon's" listings. This may include if the doctor limits their practice in any way. To find out if they are board certified or have done an otology/neurotology fellowship call their office and ask or check in "The Official ABMS Directory of Board Certified Medical Specialists" at the local library or on the Internet at www.abms.org The American Academy of Otolaryngology-Head and Neck surgery should also be able to provide names of board certified specialists in your area.

On the Internet check the American Academy of Otolaryngology-Head and Neck Surgery site at www.entnet.org (or write them at American Academy of Otolaryngology-Head and Neck Surgery, One Prince Street, Alexandria, Virginia 22314) or check the ABMS page for board certified physicians.

Sub-specialist or specialist?

Ear balance problems can be very tricky to diagnose and treat properly. Seeing someone who limits his or her practice to this demanding area can increase the chance of a happy ending. See a neurotologist if possible; it might save a bit of time and effort in the long run.

Surgeon or not?

The broad majority of people will see a surgeon for their inner ear balance problem. For many this works out fine but others might want to see a doctor with a medical background rather than a surgeon.

Don't want to go to a surgeon? It's a lot harder to find a neurologist with training in neurotology but they do exist. UCLA, Johns Hopkins, the Cleveland Clinic, Emory University, Wake Forest University, Massachusetts Eye and Ear Infirmary and the University of Pittsburgh are some examples of institutions where they can be found.

Geography

Where a person lives plays the largest part in who they see. Some entire states have no trained otologists or neurotologists.

If unhappy with a local doctor think about going out of the area, many people do. Before leaving home contact the doctor to find out if they welcome people from outside their area and if they will keep you as a patient when you return home.

Insurance

People without much money, should make sure, even double check, that a doctor is covered by their insurance plan. Check with both the insurance/billing people at the doctor's office and with the insurance company.

> **Caution:** "Balance Centers" are not certified or inspected by any organization or agency so anyone can literally call anything a balance center. A few are not even run by, or associated with, a trained otologist or neurotologist or even a board certified otolaryngologist. Check on this before going.

Why go to anyone?

Is a doctor needed at all? Maybe not, but there are some things you might miss out on by not having one.

Of course doctors have all that formal education and lots of initials at the end of their names, but beyond that they have experience in this. It only makes sense to take advantage of what they've learned from the hardships other people have suffered through. A good treatment from a doctor might just be available to get a person back on track.

Perhaps the symptoms aren't from an inner ear balance problem but instead from something else that should be treated sooner rather than later. There are an extremely tiny number of people who have something wrong that could threaten life or limb if left undiscovered and untreated.

Maybe you would benefit from prescription medications.

An insurance company is not going to pay for drugs and treatments you set up for yourself. They usually do pay for treatments ordered by a doctor.

If you are one of the minority of people who have an inner ear balance problem for a really long time you may need a paper trail for disability purposes. Neither an insurance company, nor the social security administration, is going to give out disability benefits to someone who hasn't been going regularly to a traditional health care provider. I know, this isn't fair—but it's reality.

Last, trying to treat yourself could be hazardous. After all, you can't look into your own ear(s), watch your own walking, do X-Rays or scans, prescribe drugs or do fancy tests. And if you could, would you know what you were looking at or what to do about it?

Sum Up

There are a lot of doctors involved in the diagnosis and treatment of vestibular disorders.

Next

Symptoms are covered in the next chapter.

References and Reading List:

_____. *The Official ABMS Directory of Board Certified Medical Specialists*, Vol. 3, Otolaryngologists, 32 edition. N.J.: Marquis Who's Who, 1999.

Chapter Three:
The Symptoms

Not only can inner ear balance problems cause a lot of really nasty symptoms, they can also cause some very peculiar ones.

In General
The body depends on getting movement and gravity information from the ear. When it doesn't get the right information there's he—to pay with both symptoms and problems with balance function.

What's the deal? Why so many symptoms?

It isn't just the ears making symptoms. The body responds physically and emotionally when an ear feels as if it's having a melt down.

Symptoms from ear balance problems can happen out of the blue or can come from something specific, be a mere nuisance or disabling, constant or on-again, off-again, start and stop suddenly or gradually, can go on for a short time or for years and may occur on their own or along with hearing problems and/or tinnitus and/or ear fullness.

The Symptom List
The following is a list of symptoms that can occur alone or in any combination imaginable from a vestibular disorder. The symptoms are listed alphabetically, not in order of severity.

- Anger, fear, anxiety, dread, panic, worry, feeling of doom and gloom, pounding heart, worry, cold sweat
- Blurred, bouncing and/or double vision, trouble watching motion, jerking vision, difficulty focusing, difficulty looking through binoculars, cameras, microscopes, and/or telescopes, difficulty with glare
- Clumsiness, difficulty walking, difficulty turning, feeling of walking through the floor, running into things, hanging on to things, stumbling, sudden falls, looking down while walking, staggering, feeling of being pushed, touching things while walking, sudden loss of balance, tilting, unsteadiness
- Cotton in the head or ears feeling
- Difficulty concentrating, thinking, reading, sleeping; stuttering,
- Difficulty in the dark

- Drunk feeling, nothing seems right, things seem different, uneasy feeling, unreal feeling
- Ear fullness, pain, pressure
- Fatigue
- Feelings of false movement or spinning
- Headache
- Hearing loss, ringing (tinnitus), sound distortion, sound sensitivity, inability to determine sound direction
- Lightheaded, heavy headed, hung-over, swimming/floating and/or empty headed feelings
- Loss of self-esteem, self-confidence, and/or self-reliance
- Motion intolerance and/or sickness
- Muscle stiffness, stiff neck, neck ache, trembling
- Vomiting, nausea, loss of appetite, queasiness

Caution: Just because a symptom is on the list and you have it doesn't mean you have an inner ear balance disorder. On the flip side a person with an inner ear balance disorder can also have symptoms not on the list.

The following list contains some additional symptoms that children may have.

- Always eager to please
- Clinging to a parent
- Crying
- Fear of being alone
- Fright/alarm/terror
- Ignoring the spoken word
- Not wanting to play
- Quiet and withdrawn
- Seeks reassurance
- Staggering around
- Stomachaches
- Sudden falls
- Upsets easily
- Yelling out for a parent

Some Definitions
While on the topic of symptoms I'll define a few of the terms you're bound to run into again and again in your travels. Some of these can't be found in general medical dictionaries while others are there but not described accurately or in-depth.

Dizzy and dizziness
As mentioned in "Chapter One" the words dizzy and dizziness have no exact meaning and can include any or all of a number of weird sensations; lightheadedness, faintness, movement illusions, feelings of non-reality, floating, swimming, or rocking sensations, spinning, nausea and queasiness, to name a few. Sometimes the words dizzy or dizziness really only mean symptoms are present and a person just doesn't feel normal.

Because there is no standardized use, don't use the terms during visits with health care providers—it could confuse them.

Disequilibrium (also spelled dysequilibrium)
From the medicalese this is literally translated as difficult or painful equilibrium. It's used by neurotologists to describe a vague sense of unsteadiness, imbalance, tilting or bumping into things that can occur with ear balance disorders.

Vertigo
The word vertigo came from the French word, vertige, to turn. Because of this original meaning, doctors have historically used the term to describe a sense of spinning. There has been a move away from limiting the term to spinning and this book will use the expanded Vestibular Disorders Association definition of vertigo, "Perception of movement (either of yourself or of objects around you) that is not occurring or is occurring differently from what you perceive."
Some doctors like to call the spinning type of vertigo real vertigo or true vertigo.

Proprioception
The collection and use of information about the length and motion of muscles and joints by nerves in the muscles, tendons, joints, ligaments and connective tissue that figures out body position, movement and gravity.

Sum Up
There are many different symptoms possible from a vestibular disorder. It takes much more than a list of symptoms to diagnose a vestibular problem.

Next
The structure and function of the ear, known within health care and science as anatomy and physiology, is covered in the next chapter

References and Reading List:
Bronstein, A. "Under-rated neuro-otological symptoms: Hoffman and Brookler 1978 revisited." *British Medical Bulletin,* 63:213-221, 2002.

Yardley, L. *Vertigo and Dizziness.* London: Routledge, 1994. www.menieres.co.uk/vertigo_and _dizziness.html

Chapter Four
The Workings of the Ear

Everyone knows the ear hears, some even know it has something to do with balance, but most don't know the other things it does, like its part in vision and blood pressure regulation.

Over the next few pages I'll try to unravel some of the mysteries of what the ear does and how it does it. The symptoms and strange feelings you are having might be more understandable after reading this. But before we can get started in a serious way a quick tour of the ear is needed.

Our ears are divided into three areas, the external ear, middle ear and inner ear. Only one area is involved in balance, the inner ear. Just like the ear, the inner ear is divided into three areas, the cochlea, vestibule and semicircular canals.

The cochlea is the hearing area of the inner ear and the two others are for balance. All the inner ear balance areas are referred to as the vestibular areas and their function referred to as vestibular function. So, the ear balance function is more correctly called vestibular function or inner ear balance function and I'll be using that terminology from here on in.

Now that you've had the quick tour it's time to move on to a bit more detail. I'll start with hearing because it's the easiest and fastest to describe. We'll get to balance and the other really good stuff a bit later.

Hearing

This book will only provide a basic explanation of hearing. There's much more information available in dozens of books and professional journals devoted to hearing.

The ear is designed, in part, to move sound from the air to the brain. All three of its parts: the external ear, middle ear and inner ear work to make this happen.

Sound waves are collected and funneled into the head by the external ear. Each collector flap on the side of the head is called the pinna or auricle. A tunnel called the ear canal or external auditory canal (EAC) runs from the pinna into the ear.

At the end of the canal the sound waves run right smack into the eardrum (tympanic membrane or TM). Since it blocks the end of the ear canal the eardrum vibrates when hit and this movement is passed along to the little middle ear bones attached to it and to one another. These bones cross the hollow middle ear.

First the malleus connects to both the eardrum and the incus. Then the incus hooks up with the stapes, which in turn attaches to a membrane-covered hole into the inner ear called the oval window. So, sound is collected by the pinna, funneled into the ear by the external auditory canal and then passes through the middle ear along a group of tiny bones: the malleus, incus and stapes.

As each sound vibration arrives at the eardrum it pushes the stapes slightly in and out of the oval window. One of the inner ear fluids, endolymph, is pushed so much the movement through the cochlea created by it is called the traveling wave.

Along the length of the cochlea there are little cells called hair cells with hair-like things called cilia sticking up into an endolymph filled area. The fluid movement created by sound causes these "hairs" to bend right where they sprout up from the cell surface. When they bend, a chemical change takes place that causes an information signal to be sent along the cochlear branch of the vestibulocochlear nerve to the brain.

Technical point: This bending is more correctly referred to as shearing.

A problem anywhere along the path of hearing; the external ear, middle ear, inner ear, nerve or brain; can disturb function. Infection, trauma, disease, allergy, a structural problem and bad genes can all decrease or disturb hearing in some way.

Balance
Balance, and the ear's role in it, is a bit more complicated than hearing. Because of this there are two versions, the super simple no-frills version and the longer, more detailed in-depth version.

Simple
The parts of the inner ear involved in balance are the vestibule and semicircular canals. They collect and send movement and gravity information to the brain through the vestibulocochlear nerve. Once in the brain this information, along with more from other areas of the body, is used not only for balance but also for other functions like clear vision during head movement.

When there's a problem getting and using this information in the inner ear, the vestibulocochlear nerve, or the brain, symptoms can occur, sometimes with a vengeance.

In-depth
The role of the inner ears in balance is to collect and send information about movement that is increasing or decreasing in speed to the brain. Both the vestibule and semicircular canals are in on the action. Their shape, and the design of their cells, determines the way they function and the information they are able to collect.

Vestibule
The vestibule contains two little organs, the saccule and utricle. At times these organs are collectively referred to as the otolithic organs or otoliths. Their job is to sense both acceleration in a straight line and gravity; they do not sense movement at an unchanging rate of speed.

Each contains a macula, an area covered with hair cells bathed in inner ear fluid. These hair cells are almost like those found in the cochlea with a cell body and little hair-like things, cilia, sticking up from the top surface. They are different though, because a jelly-like substance surrounds them and the tops are covered with calcium carbonate crystals.

These calcium carbonate crystals are also called otoconia and one crystal an otoconium. At times they are also called the otoliths.

Of course with the rocks on top, it's top heavy. When something causes the otoconia to move the jelly goes along but the cell bodies don't, so the hairs bend right where they stick up from the surface of the cell. When bent in one direction only, toward the largest hair, the cells send electrical signals to the brain along the vestibulocochlear nerve.

Due to the design of the macula (plural: maculae) each cell's cilia only sends a signal when bent in one direction. The brain then sorts out which hair cells had their cilia bent and determines movement or gravity change from this.

Semicircular Canals

Each ear has three semicircular canals. These semicircular canals are just like their name implies, circular, but only form 2/3 of a circle. Their job is to sense increasing and decreasing circular movement, not movement at a steady rate of speed.

Just like the hair cells of the saccule and utricle, the hair cells of the semicircular canals are grouped together in one area and don't line the entire canal. They are gathered in the crista ampullaris located in the ampulla of each canal

The "hairs" of these hair cells stick up into jelly-like stuff but unlike their cousins in the vestibule, there are no crystals. This lump of jelly is called the cupula and it runs from one wall to the other and from top to bottom within the ampulla making a watertight seal.

Only circular movement increasing or decreasing in speed can be felt by the semicircular canals. Gravity and straight movement do nothing here because there are no crystals and a measurement called the specific gravity is the same in the cupula as in the surrounding fluid.

Each canal is filled with two fluids, perilymph and endolymph.

All the canals are at right angles to each other, so head movement in any geometric plane can be felt. The fluid in the semicircular canal doesn't immediately move with the head during increasing head movement but the cupula does. As a result the cupula presses against the fluid that isn't yet moving. Because the cupula totally blocks the canal the pressure backs up causing the fluid to push into the cupula and bend the "hairs" sending a signal to the brain. The brain figures out which canal is sending information and decides what movement is occurring. The signal stops flowing once the speed is constant because the head, fluid and cupula are then all moving together.

Then What?

So, the ear collects information about gravity, straight movement that's increasing or decreasing, and circular movement that's increasing or decreasing, and sends this information on to the brain. But then what happens?

Most of the information arrives in the vestibular nuclei, which is the vestibular command center in the brain (and may also be called the vestibular nuclear complex). Here it is automatically used to help "keep your balance" by using your muscles including, moving the eyes to prevent bouncing vision, adjusting chest muscles for proper breathing and making blood pressure changes in the fractions of a second after standing up.

> **Technical point**: Some vestibular information bypasses the vestibular center of the brain and goes directly to the brain area that needs it. A full explanation of this can be found in technical books and journals.

Although this section is named balance, that title really isn't completely right. The information collected by the vestibular areas of the ear is used for much more than balance and balance needs much more than inner ear information to take place normally.

The ear doesn't work alone in balance. Many body parts must be working and the brain able to receive and act upon movement, gravity and position information for balance to occur. These body parts include: the brain, spinal cord, nerves to the arms and legs, muscles, tendons, and joints.

Three body sensory systems: vestibular, visual and proprioceptive, are also needed for the best balance (Proprioception is the collection and use of information about the length and motion of muscles and joints by nerves in the muscles, tendons, joints, ligaments and connective tissue that figures out body position, movement and gravity). Some balance can be done with only two of the systems up and running. Strong muscles, flexible joints, experience and practice are also needed for the best balance.

Once in the brain, vestibular information is used so rapidly and automatically many of the vestibular-brain exchanges are called reflexes. These reflexes include the vestibulospinal reflex (VSR), vestibulocular reflex (VOR), vestibular-cervical reflex (VCR), vestibular-phrenic, and vestibulo-autonomic reflexes.

The VSR uses vestibular information arriving in the brain to automatically send out contraction and relaxation signals to the proper muscles in the neck, trunk, arms and legs.

The VCR works in pretty much the same way but the muscle signals from this reflex go to the neck to help keep the head in proper position.

Sum Up
Optimal balance requires

- A properly working brain
- Working spinal cord and peripheral nerves
- Muscles, tendons, and joints that are strong and flexible
- Experience and practice in the activity being done
- Three sensory systems; vestibular, visual and proprioceptive

Problems with any of these, not just the ears, can affect balance.

Vision
The relationship between the ears and eyes is a pretty close one with vision needed for the best balance and vestibular information needed for the clearest vision.

Movement and Position Sense
Earlier when I said the ears don't sense movements at a constant speed you probably thought I was full of hot air, didn't you? You know when you're moving at a steady rate, don't you? Vision helps fill in this information for the brain.

Vision lets us see objects ahead become larger and larger when approached and smaller and smaller when backing away from them. The blur of objects rushing by our side (peripheral vision) also tips off the brain to motion.

In addition, vision supplies information about the location of vertical and horizontal, crucial for balance. Balance can be accomplished without vision but the brain must then rely totally on vestibular and proprioceptive information. Balance without vision is much more difficult, maybe even impossible if a vestibular problem is going on.

Clear Vision
How on earth can the ears be involved in vision? It happens through the VOR, the fastest reflex in the body. Each nerve fiber leading away from a vestibular hair cell connects the eye movement muscles through a string of three nerve cells (neurons). Imagine walking forward

and staring at something in the distance. While walking forward your head moves up and down a bit but that thing in front remains clearly visible. How can that be?

In order to see, the image of the thing you're looking at must enter the front of the eye and hit the back of it in a small area called the fovea.

To keep the image during head movement, the eye must adjust. If the eyes stayed fixed in just one position during head movement, the thing being watched would appear to bounce up and down, blur and possibly even change shape.

Instead of having bouncy vision the VOR automatically moves the eyes at the exact same speed as the head but in the other direction. When the head goes up the eyes go down, when the head moves right or left the eyes move left or right. So, the eyes will automatically move opposite to the direction of head movement at the same speed.

This function can't be carried out consciously - by the time we realize where we're moving to and how fast, it would be too late to adjust the eyes.

The VOR must work behind the scenes to move the eyes constantly, automatically and rapidly into the proper positions so we can see all the objects around us during head movement. This head movement can be the head alone like shaking the head yes or the head along with the body like when walking, running, rocking in a chair, etc.

Abnormal VOR

Vestibular disorders can disturb the VOR on one or both sides. Two different problems can occur from this, nystagmus and oscillopsia.

Nystagmus is eye jerking (that's usually considered abnormal). A reduction or loss of VOR on one side or dysfunction on one or both sides can cause nystagmus.

During nystagmus the eyes move together in one direction and then move rapidly back to the center (reset). Nystagmus can occur as one jerk, in small fast groups, or for long periods of time without stopping.

It can cause the vision to jerk or make things look like they are jumping or moving rapidly, particularly in the peripheral vision. If the nystagmus is rapid and constant surroundings can even appear to spin.

Oscillopsia is bouncing or oscillating vision. The usual cause in people with an inner ear dizziness disorder is an absent or greatly reduced VOR.

Someone missing their VOR on both sides lives in a world where everything appears to bounce and blur whenever they move their head. Two personal stories describing life without the VOR are:

J.C. "Living without a balancing mechanism." *The New England Journal of Medicine*, 246:458-460, 1952.
Campbell. P "E-4: The Way I See It." Portland, Or. Vestibular Disorders Association. 1999.

Nystagmus can come from

- Reduced or lost VOR on one side
- Total VOR loss in one ear and dysfunction in the other ear
- One sided dysfunction
- Two sided dysfunction
- Partial loss in both ears
- Some types of neurological disease (that may have nothing to do with the vestibular system)

- Reduced function in both ears

Some doctors refer to oscillopsia from an absent VOR on both sides caused by vestibular disease as Dandy's syndrome. Oscillopsia isn't the same as Dandy's syndrome because oscillopsia can occur in people who have nothing wrong with their ears.

Nystagmus and oscillopsia can both come from other problems too. Their presence does not "make" the diagnosis of an inner ear balance or dizziness disorder. Their absence also doesn't mean there isn't one.

Earlier I said that the VOR is not a true reflex. Because it isn't a true reflex we can control it a bit. An example is that nystagmus can be stopped (suppressed) at times by staring really hard at a stationary object about two feet from the face. Sometimes this can also stop the feeling of vertigo during an attack.

Sum Up

So, vision is used for balance and vestibular information is used for clear vision through the VOR. Besides being the reason many folks with vestibular disorders have visual symptoms this link between the eyes and ears is also the basis for many vestibular tests currently in use.

Other

Over the past decade basic research has discovered vestibular information isn't just used for balance and clear vision, but also for blood pressure, heart rate and breathing. This research has shown that vestibular nerve fibers travel from the inner ear to the brain areas regulating these important functions. They've also discovered in lab animals that measurable changes occur when the flow of vestibular information is stopped.

> **Relax**—Absent or disrupted vestibular information does not cause a failure of the heart, blood pressure or breathing. The broad majority of people with vestibular disorders will never be aware of the relationship between vestibular information and heart rate, blood pressure and breathing.

Vestibular information is used reflexly for blood pressure, heart rate and breathing much the same way it's used for the VOR and other vestibular reflexes. The information travels through nerve fibers from the ear to the brain and then through nerve fibers to the appropriate muscles.

In the milliseconds after standing up from a sitting position vestibular information is used to adjust blood pressure and redirect contraction and relaxation patterns of the breathing muscles.

In the case of blood pressure if there weren't any changes in the size of blood vessels when a person stood up all their blood would just fall toward their feet and the brain wouldn't have enough oxygen. Instead the vestibular-autonomic reflex comes into play. As a person stands up from a sitting position this information is sent to the brain and signals sent to the appropriate blood vessels to change in size and prevent the blood from just dropping. After the first milliseconds, yes, fractions of a second, another blood pressure regulating process, the baroreflex, takes over.

There's evidence position changes cause an increase in the depth and rate of breathing and adjustments in the chest muscles and diaphragm via the vestibulo-phrenic reflex (phrenic refers to the phrenic nerve serving the diaphragm).

Research continues on this and the vestibular affect on fear/anxiety/panic and in the future may provide information about possible relationships between vestibular function and postural hypotension (low blood pressure as a person stands up), sleep apnea and related problems.

This information connection between the vestibular system and the autonomic nervous system regulating blood pressure and heart rate may also account for some of the more uncomfortable symptoms of vestibular disorders such as fear, anxiety, doom and gloom, dry mouth, palpitations, racing heart, terror, trembling, sweating, dry mouth, blurred vision, and hyperventilation.

The autonomic nervous system is also responsible for the primitive fight or flight response to danger we all experience from time to time

For more in-depth information on this check out:

Yates, B.J. and Miller, S.D. *Vestibular Autonomic Regulation.* Boca Raton, FL: CRC Press, Inc., 1996.
The January/February 1998 issue of the Journal of Vestibular Research

Fight or Flight

When we are in danger, like when a lion is approaching us (in the wilds, not at the zoo), the autonomic nervous system helps gear us up to either run away or stay put and fight it out toe to toe. Body wide signals are sent out to release adrenaline, increase the heart rate, increase the rate and depth of breathing, increase the blood flow to the brain and muscles, speed up the metabolic rate (the general functioning speed of the body), decrease blood flow to the digestive organs, slow down urine production, and causes the mouth to go dry along with a general feeling of fear and anxiety, maybe even trembling. All occur so we can hit the ground running.

Unfortunately this also occurs in response to stress that really isn't a true danger to us.

People with vestibular disorders experience many of these fight or flight changes and sensations. They are uncomfortable and noticeable because neither running away nor fighting it out are options. Instead people are left to sort of spin their wheels in the mud.

There are two explanations for why the fight or flight response occurs in folks with vestibular disorders. First, because they're scary and stressful the symptoms of vestibular dysfunction can bring on a fight or flight reaction. Second, vestibular information is automatically shared with the autonomic nervous system and might bring on the reaction directly, much in the same way that it uses vestibular information for blood pressure regulation.

Either way, the autonomic nervous system causes some pretty uncomfortable symptoms. They can be strong enough to actually overshadow the vestibular symptoms and be the main reason for seeking treatment.

Sum Up

The ear is designed for both hearing and sensing gravity and movement (increasing or decreasing in speed). This vestibular information is used constantly for balance and clear vision and for parts of blood pressure, heart rate and breathing. When vestibular function changes or stops many problems pop up and a huge variety of symptoms can begin.

Next

Where vestibular disorders come from is covered in the next chapter.

References and Reading List:

Baloh, R.W., and Honrubia, V. *Clinical neurophysiology of the vestibular system.* Philadelphia: F.A. Davis, 1992.

Baloh, R.W., and Halmagyi, G.M. *Disorders of the vestibular system.* New York: Oxford University Press, 1996.

Campbell, P. *"E-4: The way I see it."* Portland, OR: Vestibular Disorders Association, 1999.

Herdman, S.J. *Vestibular rehabilitation.* Second edition. Philadelphia: F.A. Davis, 2000.

J.C. "Living without a balancing mechanism." *The New England Journal of Medicine,* 246:458-460, 1952.

Marieb, E.N. *Human anatomy and physiology.* Fifth edition. San Francisco: Benjamin/Cummings, 2000.

Schuknecht, H. *Pathology of the ear.* Massachusetts: Harvard University Press, 1993.

Yates, B.J., and Miller, S.D. *Vestibular autonomic regulation.* Boca Raton, FL: CRC Press, Inc., 1996.

The January/February 1998 issue of the *Journal of Vestibular Research.*

The September 1, 2000 issue of *Brain Research Bulletin*

Chapter Five
Where Do Vestibular Disorders Come From?

Just like all the other organs and systems of the body, the ear can have problems from a great many causes. People are born with problem ears, inherit bad ears or develop them along the way.

Some problems begin right in the inner ear, others come from areas bordering the ear and still others come from further away in the body. Structural problems, unlucky genes, poisoning, poor blood flow, infection, and abnormal growths are all capable of producing vestibular symptoms.

The ugly reality is that not much is really known about what causes vestibular disorders and why. Right now answering the question, "Where do these come from?" involves educated guessing more than anything else.

Probably the most common explanations for vestibular symptoms people hear from their doctors are:

- I don't know what you have or what caused it
- It must be a virus
- Some of the little ear rocks have come loose and are floating around causing symptoms
- It's all in your head

The Disorders
So, what are the names of the disorders doctors and researchers figure are causing vestibular symptoms? A quick list follows and more information follows later in the book.

Acoustic neuroma: Non-cancerous tumor of the vestibular branch of the vestibulocochlear nerve that may also involve the hearing and facial nerves. (Tumors are one of the least likely causes of vestibular problems. Despite this many MD's think about them and just to be sure you don't have one will order brain MRI's and other tests).

Arnold-Chiari Malformation Type I: A structural problem in which a part of the brain is forced into an opening in the bottom of the skull.

Bacterial labyrinthitis: Bacterial infection of the inner ear usually causing vertigo, hearing loss and possibly tinnitus (ringing in the ears).

Benign Paroxysmal Positional Vertigo (BPPV): The most common vestibular disorder, apparently caused by "ear rocks" that have come loose from the utricle and are floating around touching or leaning on very sensitive structures.

Benign Paroxysmal vertigo of childhood: Sudden, short attacks of vertigo in young children that's actually a migraine condition.

Cervical or cervicogenic vertigo: Vertigo caused by the neck.

Cholesteatoma: Middle ear mass, usually from chronic otitis media, made of cholesterol and epithelium (type of tissue) that can erode away surrounding structures.

Delayed endolymphatic hydrops: Type of endolymphatic hydrops in which the start of symptoms occurs years apart.

Disabling positional vertigo: Name for a group of symptoms thought by some doctors to be caused by vascular loop compression of the vestibulocochlear nerve.

Endolymphatic hydrops: Greater than normal amount of endolymph in the inner ear.

Enlarged vestibular aqueduct syndrome: Structural problem of the inner ear in which the vestibular aqueduct is too large.

Immune system disorders: Disorder of the body system responsible for preventing infection.

Labyrinthitis: General name for any inflammation (redness and swelling) of the inner ear.

Lyme Disease: Infection spread through dear tick bites.

Mal de Debarquement: Feeling of continuing to be on a boat after leaving the boat.

Meniere's Disease: Increase in the amount of inner ear endolymph that brings on episodes of vertigo out of the blue that last 10 minutes to 24 hours, with hearing loss and tinnitus or ear fullness/pressure and without a known cause.

Migraine associated vertigo: Vertigo caused by a migraine that may or may not include a headache.

Otosclerosis: Abnormal bone growth on the inner ear's bony covering and/or the little stapes middle ear bone.

Ototoxicity: Inner ear poisoning.

Perilymphatic Fistula (PLF): Abnormal opening between the middle and inner ears allowing the escape of perilymph into the middle ear or an abnormal opening between two areas of the inner ear.

Shingles of the ear: Viral infection of the vestibulocochlear nerve.

Superior canal dehiscence: Bone abnormality in which the superior semicircular canal is not totally covered by the temporal bone.

Syphilis of the ear: Syphilis that has spread to the inner ear.

Temporal bone fracture: Fracture of the skull bone containing the inner ear.

Vascular loop syndrome: Squeezing or compression of the vestibulocochlear nerve by a blood vessel.

Vertebrobasilar insufficiency or occlusion: Decreased blood flow to the brain, inner ear and/or vestibulocochlear nerve.

Vestibular neuronitis: Viral infection/inflammation of the vestibular branch of the vestibulocochlear nerve.

Vestibulopathy: General term for any disorder of the inner ear balance areas.

Viral labyrinthitis: Viral infection/inflammation of the inner ear.

von Hippel-Lindau disease: Genetic disease that can occasionally affect the inner ear along with other body areas.

Sum Up
There are many vestibular disorders with a wide variety of causes and some with the cause remaining unknown. All of the disorders mentioned above will be discussed in more detail later in this book.

Next
The next several chapters cover diagnosis and treatment of vestibular diseases.

Chapter Six
What Do I Have?

What do I have? This question sounds simple enough, doesn't it? But many times it's more like the $64,000 question!

Up until the 1860's the symptoms we now know are caused by inner ear disorders were considered brain problems with names like apoplectic brain congestion. Back then they just didn't know the inner ear could cause so many symptoms and problems. Coming up with a diagnosis or explanation for the symptoms was all based on beliefs, assumptions and guessing, sometimes wild guessing.

Since that time making a diagnosis has become a bit more scientific but there are still many times when the best a doctor can do is point to the vestibular system in general as the culprit, not which part or why.

Luckily not having a diagnosis and explanation for the illness won't mean you can't get better or back to your old self. If your symptoms have just begun try not to get hung up on a quest for THE name before accepting a treatment. Since many of the treatments are the same no matter what the cause a lot of time, money and energy might be wasted looking for a diagnosis while gaining very little in return. As odd as it sounds, having a diagnosis doesn't always mean there's a cure or successful treatment waiting and not having a diagnosis does not mean you are doomed.

Why Is Diagnosis Such a Problem?
Vestibular disorders aren't understood all that well and there is no slam-dunk sort of test to diagnose them.

Why? Good question.

The inner ear is tiny and buried in the thickest, hardest bone of the body. It's insides can't be seen on an X-ray, MRI (Magnetic resonance imaging) or any other tests and the inner ear can't be cut open for a look inside without risking permanent hearing loss or damage to balance function.

It's just plain difficult to know a whole lot about an organ that can't be looked in or at, with function that can't be directly measured.

A lot of what we do know about the inner ear comes from animal research. This isn't a perfect situation because there are differences between people and other animals. Animals also can't describe what they are experiencing and don't seem to develop the same vestibular disorders as humans.

Human ears can be studied closely—the catch is not until after a person has died. One human research approach is studying the ears of people who had vestibular symptoms during their lives. It's assumed the changes found in their ears actually caused their problems during life. Treatments are then developed for living people and researchers try to study this more fully by creating these changes in lab animals. Unfortunately if the change didn't cause the disorder no useful knowledge is gained. Not only that, but bad information may be collected instead.

Ear, nose and throat surgeons with very little training in their diagnosis and treatment usually treat vestibular disorders. Few doctors limit their practice to vestibular disorders.

The current balance testing is very sophisticated and requires an understanding of engineering, something many doctors haven't studied.

There's more and more evidence inner ear problems can come from outside the ear, possibly even from a body-wide problem. Not all ENT's know about advances in non-ear areas of medicine and how they might apply to the ear.

Hearing gets most of the ear research dollars—sometimes vestibular information is discovered during hearing research but it's only luck when that happens, not a well thought out plan.

No national or international vestibular organization exists to direct and raise funds for research.

All of this adds up to trouble, not only is the diagnosis of vestibular disorders difficult but so to is their treatment. Unlike many other diseases, vestibular disorders are categorized by their symptoms, not by how they damage the body or it's function. Usually a doctor casually notices that they've seen a particular set of symptoms in their patients. If the symptom pattern occurs in enough people the doctor may write about it in a medical journal and refer to it with a name of some sort. If a physical change is found in the ears of one or two of these people after they've died it's assumed everyone with this symptom pattern has the same change. Assumed is the key word here because tests of vestibular function just can't find these changes in living people.

This means diagnosis, treatment and research are usually based on a string of assumptions, not scientifically supported truths.

How Will Your Doctor Figure Out What You Have?

They'll hear your story, do an examination and probably order some tests. Doctors must collect a lot of information and piece it together like a puzzle hoping to understand what the picture shows in the end.

Coming up with a diagnosis can be almost like the process a prosecutor goes through to set up a circumstantial evidence case for a trial. One shred of evidence won't lead to a conviction but a pile of it might. But just like in a court some doubt will exist in the absence of an eyewitness or some sort of direct, physical evidence.

Sum Up

Understanding and diagnosing vestibular problems is difficult at best.

Next

The next three chapters cover the history, examination and testing for vestibular disorders. Later in the book individual vestibular disorders will be done.

Chapter Seven
The History

The most crucial step in figuring out what's wrong and determining a treatment is hearing the full story. What's being experienced now? When did it start? What makes it worse? Does anything help it? Without this sort of information even $10,000 worth of tests most likely won't produce an accurate diagnosis.

If the doctor you see doesn't want to listen to your story don't waste time with them. Listening to a history isn't polite; it's crucial for an appropriate diagnosis. Without this information they can't formulate a working diagnosis, determine the appropriate tests needed or design a personalized treatment plan. Get yourself someone who will listen.

Giving a History

If you have trouble thinking and speaking it might be a good idea to get your story or history organized before seeing a doctor for the first time. This way there's less chance of leaving anything out or giving a confused story that a doctor might be unable to follow.

Doctor's are only human and may not be able to stay completely attentive during long stories filled with flowery descriptions accented with private theories and other information. Try to keep to the facts, if feeling lightheaded say so plainly and clearly, don't launch into your theories of where it's coming from—unless asked for these additional details. Keep it short, sweet and accurate; don't leave anything out but stay on topic and don't meander.

If experiencing violent spinning say that and not that its the worst spinning ever visited upon a human being since the beginning of time and you feel like you're being hurled into space and lost forever in a dark vortex of horror.

Stay away from one-word descriptions like vertigo, nystagmus or oscillopsia. If having episodes of spinning say that, don't call it vertigo. Be sure your doctor knows exactly what you mean. Their definition of vertigo, nystagmus or oscillopsia may differ from yours. If your vision is bouncing say that. Don't ever assume your definition is the same as theirs.

Should you walk into an appointment with a printed history? Good question. Some doctors have a questionnaire for you to fill out, so writing out something ahead of time could prove a waste of time and effort. If they don't have a questionnaire, your own written summary would be helpful.

On the other hand some doctors might feel intimidated by this or feel your real problem is being wrapped up in concerns about your body and that nothing "real" is wrong or that you are blowing something small all out of proportion.

You'll have to decide for yourself how to handle this. Go with the clarity and organization of a written document or take a small gamble that the doctor will think you really aren't sick at all and it's all in your head.

What They Usually Want to Know About the Symptoms:

- What are the symptoms?
- When did they begin?
- Has this happened before?
- What was happening when first experienced?
- Are they always the same or do they increase or decrease?
- What causes them to increase or decrease?
- Does anything stop them?
- Do they come in episodes?
- How severe are they?
- Do the symptoms stay the same? Increase or decrease?
- Any drugs being taken or special diet eaten?
- The general health of blood relatives
- Are nausea and vomiting present?
- Is there tinnitus or a hearing loss?
- Sensitivity to sounds of any sort?

If You Are Having Attacks:

- Does anything seem to bring them on?
- Any ear infections in the past?
- Do relatives have similar symptoms now, or in the past?
- Any allergies or hay fever now or in the past?
- Ever had migraines?
- The treatments and diets being used
- Have antibiotics been used recently? Before the symptoms began?

Sum Up
Giving your doctor an accurate and thorough history is the first and most important step on the way to a diagnosis. It's every bit as important as an examination or any test.

Next
The next chapter covers the examination.

References and Reading List:
McNaboe, E., and Kerr, A. "Why history is the key in the diagnosis of vertigo." *Practitioner,* 244(1612):648-653, 2000.

Rosenberg, M.L., and Gizzi, M. "Neuro-otologic history." *Otolaryngologic Clinics of North America, 33(3):471-482, 2000.*

Chapter Eight
The Examination

The next step after giving a history is an examination. This, coupled with the history, may give your doctor enough information to make a diagnosis. If not, the examination should help in figuring out what tests are needed to make one.

Before seeing a specialist visit a primary care provider (PCP) for a general once over. The inner ears aren't the only place dizziness can come from. Let them look for problems they can explain, diagnose and treat. A PCP might be able to figure out what's wrong or at least what's not wrong. This can help in determining if a specialist should be seen and if so, who.

> **Note:** Since this is an inner ear book this chapter is limited to what an examination of inner ear balance function might include. It doesn't contain information about examinations of the cardiovascular and neurological systems.

Before I Go On, a Warning:
Showing How You Feel

A person might think since their symptoms and problems can't be seen they will be ignored or not taken seriously. Some people may even feel their problems have already been ignored or downplayed by members of the health care professions. As a result they may not try their hardest during tests of balance or might even allow themselves to fall so their problems can be seen.

Don't try to show a doctor how you feel. An attempt to show symptoms of balance and vestibular dysfunction can lead to the wrong diagnosis, or worse, make them think nothing is physically wrong. It might sound odd, but falling and visibly poor balance are not always present in a vestibular disorder.

Tell your doctor about your symptoms and problems, don't try to show them. If they don't take them, or you, seriously, move on to someone who will.

The Examination

What the examination consists of has a lot to do with the type specialist you see. An otolaryngologist may begin with a general ear, nose and throat exam including looking in the nose and at the vocal cords in addition to looking in the ears. An otologist or neurologist may stay entirely focused on the ear checking hearing, the external ear and balance function. A neurologist specializing in dizziness might spend more time looking at the function of the neurological system. Although they differ, neither approach is wrong or bad.

A thorough exam by any of these specialists should include checks of the:

- Ear
- Hearing
- Brain and nervous system (selected areas)
- Balance and movement
- Eye movement

Obviously the purpose of the exam is to find out what's wrong so something can be done about it. If a vestibular disorder is suspected a specialist will look for both abnormalities in function and absence of function before coming to a conclusion about the diagnosis and making a decision about how to proceed next.

Caution: When going for an examination wear something comfortable and take someone along who can help you get home-on occasion this type examination can bring on a temporary increase in symptoms or the temporary appearance of new ones.

Ear
The external ear canal can be checked for infection, wax buildup, the presence of a foreign body, and holes in the eardrum. They can also check for middle ear fluid, infection and an ear growth called a cholesteatoma.

Hearing
Hearing should definitely be checked. It will either be done by the doctor with tuning forks or in a sound proof booth by an audiologist (or both). The sound proof booth is the only way to accurately test hearing.

Brain and Nervous System
Because some brain and nervous system diseases can also cause symptoms similar to those of vestibular disorders, a very limited exam of their function is done.

Eye movement, pupil reaction to light, the inside of the eyes, the ability to touch the nose with an index finger, facial muscle movement, movement coordination, how a person walks, how their senses are functioning and the ability to answer questions are all checked.

In the unlikely chance there's a problem in any of these areas a neurologist will be recommended.

Balance and Movement
Several tests of balance consisting of variations in standing and walking can be done during an office exam.

One of the oldest tests in use is the Romberg in which you stand quietly with arms at your sides (or possibly held straight out in front) and feet side by side with your eyes open and then closed. Try to relax during the Romberg test. The doctor will be right there to catch you in the unlikely event you should start to fall.

A more modern addition to the test may also be done by standing with one foot in front of the other, toes of one foot touching the heel of the other, with arms folded across the chest, eyes open and then eyes closed. They also might give a gentle push during the test.

They'll also want to see you walk, perhaps with your eyes closed and sometimes walking heel to toe, one foot in front of the other. They might ask you to walk or march in place and to turn rapidly while walking.

Eye Movement
The eyes will be observed for nystagmus (eye jerking) while staring at the finger of the examiner or at a light and may also be observed while moving the head. In addition they may look for nystagmus while you move your head back and forth or when the examiner moves it. They may also watch for it while you cough or strain.

The examiner may also move the head rapidly while staring at the face and may perform a Dix-Hallpike test to see if a very specific, rapid position change brings on nystagmus and vertigo. To be useful, the Dix-Hallpike must be done in a specific manner. Directions must be followed completely and the positions maintained as instructed no matter what symptoms occur.

Sum Up
In addition to collecting a history your doctor will do an examination. This examination will look at many functions and body areas to determine both what isn't wrong and what might be wrong. Exams differ from doctor to doctor but as a bare minimum should include the areas described in this chapter.

Next
Testing will be covered in the next chapter.

References and Reading List:
Baloh, R.W., and Halmagyi, G.M. *Disorders of the vestibular system.* New York: Oxford University Press, 1996.

Goebel, J.A. *Practical management of the dizzy patient.* Philadelphia: Lippincott Williams & Wilkins, 2001.

Shepard, N.T., and Telian, S.A. *Practical management of the balance disorder patient.* San Diego, CA: Singular Publishing Group, 1996.

Chapter Nine
Testing

For many people testing is the last step on the road to a diagnosis. In most cases testing can't be used alone to make a conclusive diagnosis but will help build up evidence for the presence of one disorder or the absence of another.

Tests can be used to help determine the treatment, and be used over time to see if a person is improving, staying the same or getting worse. When the ear causing the problem isn't known, testing might help in finding out.

Several types of tests are in use including: balance, blood, eye movement, hearing, imaging and vision tests.

Before Going For Any Tests:

Some tests are surprisingly expensive. It's crucial to have the proper insurance authorization before undergoing any tests. If paying for the test out of your own pocket, check on the prices first to avoid a nasty surprise later.

Ask the testing center or doctor's office for test instructions. They might ask you to stop taking certain drugs a day or two before the test and may have some other instructions too. Wear a comfortable pair of slacks, shorts or sweatpants when going for vestibular testing and have a ride home arranged.

DO NOT drive yourself home if the tests have increased your symptoms or you are experiencing sudden, spontaneous attacks of vertigo without any warning.

> **Note:** In this chapter I'll use the word tester for the person conducting the test and testee for the person undergoing the test.

Balance

The computerized dynamic posturography test (CDP) is a sophisticated test of standing balance. It's also called dynamic posturography, moving platform posturography, dynamic computerized platform posturography and platform posturography.

It tests the vestibulospinal reflex and can help figure out if a balance problem is coming from the inner ear or the brain. It can also be used over time to track a person's progress and to help in designing an individualized treatment plan. One drawback: this test isn't real useful in trying to determine which ear is the problem and may only indicate the presence of a vestibular disorder, not which problem.

The CDP system in most widespread use is the Equitest. Testing is divided into a couple of parts, the sensory organization test (SOT), the motor coordination test (MCT) and the optional pressure test. Quiet standing balance is measured in the SOT; MCT measures the testee's reflex response when the bottom of the apparatus is moved and the pressure test measures standing balance while the air pressure is changed in the ear canals. Some doctors also add their own little parts to the test such as moving or holding the head in different positions. A bill for this test may not list computerized dynamic posturography but instead list individual components such as the sensory organization test, muscle coordination test or pressure test.

The testee stands on the surface of the test machine with a colored wall in front and on both sides. All that's required of the testee is to stand exactly where the tester places them and follow their directions, i.e. when to open or close their eyes. The wall or floor of the apparatus may move at times but the testee is asked not to change the position of their feet or move around. Since it's a standing test a safety harness is used to prevent injury if a fall should occur.

The sensory organization part of the test is designed to figure out how well balance is maintained when information comes from all three sensory systems (vestibular, vision and proprioception), just 2 systems or from only 1 system.

> **Note:** Proprioception is the collection and use of information about the length and motion of muscles and joints by nerves in the muscles, tendons, joints, ligaments and connective tissue. This information is used by the brain to figure out body position, movement and gravity. Sometimes it's also referred to as somatosensory function.

At times the motor coordination test can help in figuring out if it's the inner ear or the brain causing a balance problem. The pressure test may be useful in the diagnosis of perilymphatic fistula.

Blood Tests

Of course there is no slam-dunk blood test to detect the presence of a vestibular disorder. (If there were you wouldn't need this book) A few blood tests can uncover conditions that are capable of causing vestibular problems or symptoms like syphilis, hypothyroidism, allergies, Lyme disease, high cholesterol and autoimmune disorders. A blood test for syphilis is important because it's still a common disease and, more important, it can be successfully treated at times.

Sometimes blood is sent to distant labs for special virus and antibody tests. None of these tests can prove, on their own, that the ear is being bothered by any of these culprits or which ear might be under attack. Some, like those for autoimmune disorders and Lyme disease, can't prove anything, but can raise suspicion.

For example, testing may show hypothyroidism but that doesn't prove the thyroid is causing the vestibular symptoms. It might just mean that in addition to having a vestibular problem there's a thyroid problem.

Results of blood tests are added to all the other bits and pieces of information collected to see if evidence is mounting for a particular diagnosis.

Don't assume your doctor isn't being thorough if no exotic blood tests have been done, it could be they just don't suspect anything that can be confirmed by blood tests or feel blood tests are too iffy to help (of course it's also possible they aren't being thorough).

Eye Movement

So, what does eye movement have to do with anything? Because the eyes and ears are tied closely together via the vestibulocular reflex it's not surprising there are tests to check VOR function.

These tests aren't a sure thing. They're only one piece of evidence, not the whole enchilada. Sometimes they'll only show there's a problem, not which one.

Note: For extremely in-depth technical information about all aspects of eye movement check out: Leigh, R.J., Zee, D.S. *The neurology of the eye movements.* Third edition. Philadelphia: F.A. Davis company, 1999.

Go for this testing wearing something comfortable. Don't wear make-up around your eyes. If you have a blind eye or other serious visual problem tell them ahead of time. Be sure to make arrangements for someone to drive you home after the test.

To observe and record eye movements all the tests are done with either infrared goggles over the eyes or with sticky electrodes pasted on the face. Blinking can interfere with the test and should be avoided if at all possible.

ENG

The electronystagmogram or ENG is the most common test done in people suspected of having a vestibular disorder. Almost everyone with the diagnosis of a vestibular disorder has had it done, or I should say, them. The ENG is really a series of tests done in succession over roughly an hour and as such will usually show up on a bill as a series of separate tests.

Eye movement is observed, recorded and measured during the test.

Although nystagmus is in its name much of the ENG has little to do with nystagmus. Not all of the ENG tests look for vestibular disease either. Instead they check eye movements controlled by different areas of the brain.

The series of tests can include:

- Caloric
- Fistula or pressure
- Gaze
- Head shaking
- Optokinetic after-nystagmus
- Optokinetic nystagmus
- Positional
- Positioning (Dix-Hallpike)
- Saccades
- Smooth Pursuit
- Spontaneous nystagmus
- Visual tracking

During testing the testee sits in a chair or on a table with the tester right next to them. They're asked to follow moving lights with their eyes, look at stationary lights, move their head, change their position, and might have their head moved by the tester. In the last part of the test warm and cool water or air are inserted into the ear canal.

Of all the tests in the ENG the caloric is the one people remember the most. This test stimulates the vestibular organs and records the eye response. It's done lying down with the head elevated a bit. The tester gently and carefully inserts a soft tube into the ear canal. Warm and cold water are then passed through the tube. (Some test facilities use air instead).

During this time the testee is asked to name names or do simple math. As silly as this seems it must be done with gusto for the test to be accurate. Keeping testees alert and preventing them from holding (fixing) their eyes in one position during the test is crucial.

Once the temperature change is underway eye movement is recorded. The NORMAL response IS spinning vertigo with nystagmus. The strength of the spinning is related to the amount of vestibular function present in the ear being tested. FEELING VERTIGO AND HAVING NYSTAGMUS IS NORMAL. The absence of vertigo and nystagmus is abnormal and can occur when there's reduced vestibular function, the tester did a poor job or a technical problem occurred.

The temperature change doesn't last long and then the testee is asked to stare straight ahead at a light or object. Fixing the vision on one spot like this almost always stops the strong vertigo.

Nystagmus occurring with the vertigo is observed, measured and recorded. A mathematical formula is used to compare the reaction of the two ears. The test measures the eye movement, not the degree of vertigo or discomfort.

> **Technical point**: If an ear doesn't respond to the warm or cool temperature change during the test icy water is then used. Whether or not this is uncomfortable depends on the amount of icy water used. Rotational testing should be done if an ENG shows no VOR function on either side. (See rotational testing below)

Unfortunately a normal ENG doesn't mean the vestibular system is normal, it just means nothing recordable was happening when the test was done or if something is wrong the ENG can't measure it. This test can only look at the function of the lateral semicircular canal which is just 1/5 of the vestibular system.

The test can help in identifying which side is the problem but can't tell if the problem is in the ear, the vestibulocochlear nerve or the brain. Some types of ENG results can lead to a specific diagnosis with a treatment while others can only point to the vestibular system in general. The problem part of the system: ear, nerve or brain, might not even be discovered.

In addition to looking at vestibular function the ENG also looks at other eye movement systems and might help in determining if a neurological disorder is the problem rather than the inner ear.

Rotation

All rotational tests take a hard look at the VOR (Vestibulocular reflex), specifically the horizontal VOR (back and forth eye movement). Some tests, such as the VAT or VORTEQ, can also look at the vertical VOR (up and down eye movement). They all take advantage of the fact that a normally functioning vestibular system will move the eyes in one direction as the head moves in the other at the same speed. All the tests are computerized and either involve moving the chair a testee is seated on at a very specific speed and direction or having the testee move their own head at a specific speed and direction. These tests are best at seeing if something is wrong in general but not at figuring out what.

Wear something comfortable for this test, have someone drive you home after the test(s) and if you are blind in an eye or have some other major vision problem call up the test center before going for the test and let them know about it.

Chair (Sometimes called the rotary chair)

The rotational chair test is usually done in a small, lightless booth—if you have claustrophobia discuss it with the testing center before making your appointment.

The testee is seated in a chair that moves at times. While the chair moves the eye response is recorded and the tests' computer software program compares chair movement to eye movement. This information is then used to measure VOR function. The testee is asked to name names or do math during different parts of the test.

The test results are very technical and compare chair speed to eye speed. The eyes should move at roughly the same time and at the same rate of speed as the chair.

VORTEQ and Vestibular Autorotation Testing (VAT)

In both these tests the testee is seated on an unmoving chair and asked to stare at something while they move their head back and forth or up and down for seconds at a time. Either a headband will be placed around the head and electrodes on the face or a pair of goggles placed on the face. The head movement and eye movement are measured and compared to determine if they are moving in sync. This testing is different from the rotational chair because they're done at a higher speed and look at the vertical VOR in addition to the horizontal VOR.

Hearing

Tests of hearing are a standard part of the vestibular workup. Hearing is checked because the cochlea is housed in the inner ear along with the vestibular structures and some disorders will affect both hearing and balance. Also, the nerve carrying hearing information to the brain also carries vestibular information. Because some vestibular disorders include hearing loss and others don't, hearing tests can help rule out some diseases or make some disorders look more likely.

People having vestibular symptoms whenever they hear loud sounds or undergo pressure changes should make arrangements for someone to drive them home after the test.

An audiologist or audiology technician generally does the tests of hearing. There are many hearing tests available. In this chapter I'm only going to cover those most commonly given to people suspected of having vestibular disorders. Many good books describing all the hearing tests in great detail are available for people who want more in-depth information.

> **Technical point:** An audiologist has completed five or six years of college studying hearing, hearing tests, and devices to aid hearing. They have earned a master's degree and passed a standardized test to become a certified audiologist with the initials CCC-A behind their name. They know more about hearing than any other licensed health care professional. An audiology technician who has less training and education may also perform hearing tests.

Pure Tone Audiology
(PTA)

Standardized single tones at various pitches and levels of loudness are played through headphones in this test and the testee is asked to let the tester know when they hear them. The results are charted on a graph showing the pitch along one line and the decibel (loudness) level on the other.

Sometimes, for technical reasons, the audiologist may add a sound device behind the ear and/or the sound of static to the test.

Speech

There are two speech tests in common use, the speech reception threshold test and word recognition test. Both are done while wearing headphones and repeating words spoken by the audiologist.

Speech reception threshold (SRT)

This test is designed to find out what loudness is needed for a person to recognize 50% of the words spoken to them. Familiar, two syllable words like cowboy and hotdog are spoken at a very quiet level, increasing in loudness until 50% of the words can be identified correctly. The test results report the level of that loudness, also called the decibel level.

Word recognition (Speech discrimination)

The aim is just what the title of the test says, word recognition. Phonetically balanced, single syllable words are spoken at 40 decibels of loudness above the speech reception threshold and the correct percentage of words identified is recorded.

Immittance audiometry tests

This group of tests checks middle ear function, eardrum movement and the acoustic reflex. They are used to rule out middle ear and eustachian tube dysfunction as the cause of vestibular symptoms. They're all done by inserting a soft plug into the ear canal connected to a computerized machine that sends either pressure or sound into the ear and measures their effect on the ear.

Tympanogram

The testee sits quietly and does nothing during this test. Positive, then negative pressure along with sound are sent into the external ear canal. Tympanic membrane (ear drum) movement is measured and printed on a graph. The shape is then interpreted to determine how well the middle ear and eustachian tube are functioning. Different conditions result in differing shapes on the graph and these shapes have letter names like Type A and Type B.

A normal tympanogram is thought to mean the eardrum is moving normally and the eustachian tube is letting atmospheric pressure into the middle ear.

Abnormalities that can be discovered with a tympanogram include a flaccid or floppy ear drum, middle ear fluid, a scarred or thickened ear drum, perforated ear drum (hole in the ear drum) ossicular discontinuity (the little ear bones are no longer connected), glue ear, otosclerosis, and ear canal occlusion.

Stapedial Reflex

This test measures the acoustic reflex and is always done after the tympanogram. The acoustic reflex causes the middle ear's stapedius muscle to contract when loud sound is heard. This muscle contraction causes the little middle ear bones to tighten up in an effort to stop all the loud sound from entering the inner ear.

In this test a sound is played through the headphones and the amount of sound sent back from the tympanic membrane measured. It's used primarily for diagnosing problems of hearing rather than vestibular disorders although folks with Meniere's disease sometimes have an odd result.

Central nervous system depressants, including alcohol can make the test inaccurate.

Auditory evoked responses

These tests measure the electrical activity created during hearing. A computer is used to send sound into the ear and interpret the electrical events from the vestibulocochlear nerve to the brain. There are two commonly used in a vestibular work-up, the ECOG and the ABR. A third, the otoacoustic emmissions test is also growing in popularity.

Auditory Brainstem Response (ABR)

The ABR is also called a BAER (brainstem auditory response), BSER (Brainstem evoked response) and a number of other similar things. It's done to measure the nerve activity of sound as it moves to the brain.

In this test electrodes are placed on the head and ear lobes or inserted into the ear canals, sounds are then played through headphones and the electrical waves they produce recorded with a computer.

The electrical activity is displayed as waves with a total of 7 produced as sound moves from the ear to the brain and then within the brain. The first wave occurs in the ear and is studied in even greater detail in the next test, the electrocochleogram, ECOG.

The ABR is usually done to check for the presence of an acoustic neuroma, a rare tumor of the vestibulocochlear nerve.

Electrocochleography (ECOG)

This test is similar to the ABR (see above) but takes a closer look at the first two waves of the ABR that occur in the cochlea and along the vestibulocochlear nerve. It's thought this can show information about the hair cells of the cochlea and can determine if there's an increased amount of endolymph in the inner ear.

Again, electrodes, sticky pads connected to wires, are placed on the head and ear lobes and soft tubes inserted into the ear canals, clicking sounds played through head phones and the electrical waves they produce recorded and analyzed with a computer. A ratio of the SP to AP is calculated during the test. If it's greater than normal it's thought there's too much of the inner ear fluid endolymph present.

Note: ECOG can't be done in a totally deaf or severely hearing impaired ear.

There are usually three parts to the test, the cochlear microphonics (CM), summating potential (SP) and the action potential (AP). A bill might list these individual tests rather than the word electrocochleogram.

Otoacoustic Emissions

This test checks on the condition of its hair cells. Yes, the ears have actually been found to make sounds both on their own and after outside sound enters the ear.

A padded soft wire containing a microphone is inserted into the ear canal for this test. Sound is sent into the ear, a microphone picks up sound made by the cochlea in response and a computer then analyzes the sound.

The test can be used to discover noise damage or cochlear poisoning before a hearing loss can be measured and can also help in hearing aid evaluation.

Even more information about hearing tests can be found in audiology books like "Essential Audiology for Physicians" by Cathleen Campbell, published by Singular Publishing Group, Inc, San Diego, CA.

Imaging Tests

Simple X-Rays of the ear are seldom done these days. Instead computerized tests like the MRI (magnetic resonance imaging) and CT (computerized tomography), capable of taking numerous "pictures," are used. None of these tests can show the insides of the inner ear or if it's working but can show the external areas of the inner ear, the vestibulocochlear nerve and the brain.

Special: If you are pregnant or might be or are trying to be, please tell both your doctor and the test facility. X-Rays can damage unborn children.

Computerized tomography (CT)

A CT is a computerized method of taking a series of X-Rays, usually done to look at bone. In the case of the ear this means looking at the temporal bone for problems like a break, wearing away of the bone, abnormal anatomy, bony defects, a tumor, cyst, or the relatively newly discovered inner ear problem, dehiscence of the superior semicircular canal.

For this test a person lays down on a table and the table is slid slowly into the CT machine where pictures are taken over a short period of time. Staying absolutely still when told to is crucial during this test.

If movement, bright lights or lying on your back stir up your symptoms plan for someone to drive you home after the test.

Magnetic Resonance Imaging (MRI)

Carefully read over the literature from the testing center before going for this test. DO NOT enter the test room until certain it's safe to do so. People with metal in their bodies, including a cochlear implant, can't have an MRI.

> **Important:** If you are susceptible to claustrophobia discuss this with the testing center before making your appointment since these computerized tests involve being placed into a small cave-like area. An MRI in a more open machine might be possible with advance planning.

When going for the test, a person should arrange for someone to take them home in case the test procedure stirs up symptoms. Wear clothing that is comfortable and easy to remove. Don't take too many belongings along because they must be left behind in a locker.

During the test you'll lay down, have your head secured so it won't move and be slid inside the machine. When the machine is running it will make a loud banging noise. If they don't give you earplugs before starting the test insist on them. One testing sequence will be done and then an IV injection of gadolinium given and the test repeated. Gadolineum is given to help identify any abnormal growths present. Let the tech know if you have poor veins or if one arm is better than the other.

This test looks at soft tissue (anything that isn't bone) using a magnetic field instead of X-Rays. A doctor may order an MRI of the brain, the inner ear areas or both. It's generally done to look for tumors, multiple sclerosis, damage from a brain attack (stroke), hydrocephalus (water on the brain) and Arnold-Chiari malformation type I and other exotic problems. A doctor usually orders up this test to be absolutely sure a person doesn't have them and not because they expect to find them. An inner ear MRI can help diagnose enlarged vestibular aqueduct or vestibular neuritis when present.

This test uses magnetism rather than X-Rays and has a different set of precautions, etc. to worry about. Anyone with objects in their body that can be moved with a magnet is excluded from having this test. These objects include cochlear implants, pacemakers, surgical clips and pins, metal shrapnel, or bullets. BE VERY CAREFUL ON THIS POINT—movement of metal within the body can cause injury, even death. Think at least twice before answering no.

The entire testing sequence must be completed for the images to be made by the computer, don't stop the test in the middle unless it's a real emergency.

Vestibular Evoked Myogenic Potentials (VEMP)
This newer test is used to determine how well the utricle is working in sensing both increasing/decreasing movement in a straight line and gravity.

Electrodes are placed on the neck and wrists and instructions given to reposition the head while sound is sent into the external auditory canal. A computer then measures the electrical muscle response.

Vision
Dynamic visual acuity testing is done to check on vision during head movement. It can be done by simply trying to read a vision or Snellen chart while moving the head back and forth or up and down or might be done as a computerized test.

The computerized version is done with a headband sensor in place while looking at a computer screen and moving the head in time with a computer generated beeping sound. While moving the head the testee is asked to say which way the open side of a square is facing.

Vision will not be as accurate in a person with a damaged VOR as it is in someone with a normal VOR.

General Problems With Tests

- They are expensive
- Some people find them quite uncomfortable and tiring
- They can seem scary
- They are technically difficult to perform and interpret—people doing them and interpreting them need lots of training and must have ongoing education
- Most lack standardization and are done so differently from one facility to another that neither the raw data nor the interpretation is usually accepted by other health care professionals
- None of the tests can see inside the inner ear
- No test can measure the electrical signals moving directly from the vestibular areas of the inner ear to the brain (there is no vestibular equivalent of the ABR test)
- Many can't differentiate between a vestibular ear problem, nerve problem or brain problem
- They don't always help in determining which ear is the problem
- Most vestibular tests only look at a very small area of the inner ear, not the whole thing

Even with all these problems they can be helpful in both the diagnosis and treatment of vestibular disorders and can be worth both the expense and bother.

Sum Up
Very few vestibular disorders can be diagnosed solely with testing. Sometimes the best a test can do is confirm something is wrong but may not be able to determine what. For more in-depth information about balance testing check out: Jacobson, G.P., Newman, C.W., and Kartush, J.M. "Handbook of balance function testing." San Diego: Singular Publishing Group, Inc. 1997

Next
Treatment is covered in the next few chapters.

References and Reading List:
Baloh, R.W., and Honrubia, V. *Clinical neurophysiology of the vestibular system.* Third edition. Oxford: Oxford University Press, 2001.

Baloh, R.W., and Halmagyi, G.M. *Disorders of the vestibular system.* Oxford: Oxford University Press, 1996.

Colebatch, J.G., Halmagyi, G.M., and Skuse, N.F. "Myogenic potentials generated by click-evoked vestibulocollic reflex." *Journal of Neurology, Neurosurgery, and Psychiatry,* 57(2):190-197, 1994.

De Waele, C. "VEMP Induced by High Level Clicks." *Advances in Otorhinolaryngology,* 58:98-109, 2001.

Ferber-Viart C., Dubreuil C., and Duclaux R. "Vestibular evoked myogenic potentials in humans: a review." *Acta Otolaryngologica,* 119:6-15, 1999.

Goebel, J.A. *Practical management of the dizzy patient.* Philadelphia: Lippincott William & Wilkins, 2001.

Kemp, D.T. "Otoacoustic emissions, their origin in cochlear function, and use." *British Medical Bulletin,* 63:223-241, 2002.

Jacobson, G.P., Newman, C.W., and Kartush, J.M. *Handbook of balance function testing.* San Diego: Singular Publishing Group, Inc., 1997.

Li, M.V., Houlden, D., and Tomlinson, R.D. "Click evoked EMG responses in sternocleidomastoid muscles: characteristics in normal subjects." *Journal of Vestibular Research,* 9(5):327-334, 1999.

Mark, A.S., and Fitzgerald, D. "MRI of the inner ear." *Baillieres Clinical Neurology,* 3(3):515-535, 1994.

Shepard, N.T., and Telian, S.A. *Practical management of the balance disorder patient.* San Diego: Singular Publishing Group, 1996.

Chapter Ten
Treatment

What can be done for vestibular disorders? In a word: lots. No matter what the diagnosis, even if there isn't one, there are treatments around including diet change, medication, physical therapy, surgery and alternative treatments such as acupuncture that may help to some degree. Unfortunately, some disorders are chronic by nature and may not totally disappear.

Finding the right treatment can be pretty fast and easy or a long, drawn out ordeal or anything in-between.

Don't make the mistake of thinking that having a diagnosis leads to a treatment that results in a cure. It might not. The opposite is also true; treatments can be quite successful even if there is no solid diagnosis.

Doctors determine the treatment through their experience, gut feelings and instincts; what they were taught in school, the published research findings they've read, the research they've heard about at medical conferences and what they are comfortable with. They also base it on the damage and symptoms along with THEIR vision of your future. Because human beings are involved in this process selecting a treatment is far from perfect and involves a whole lot more than science.

Treatments can be aimed at:

- Stopping the progression of a disease
- Reversing the changes a disease has caused
- Stopping the secondary problems created
- Reversing the secondary changes created
- Blocking the symptoms of the primary or secondary problems
- Any combination of these

A person with a vestibular disorder agrees to undergo a treatment based on a lot of factors too, including how much they trust the doctor, if the treatment seems to make sense, how much effort the treatment requires, how much discomfort the treatment brings, if the treatment is the same as they've read or heard about from other people, if they can afford the treatment itself or the time off from work it might require and simply their gut reaction to it.

The problems and symptoms to be treated can come from the disease itself or from the changes the disease or trauma have created. What your symptoms are from and what treatment is appropriate for them at a particular point in time can be a complicated puzzle to solve. It can take a really well educated and experienced neurotologist to sort through it all and come up with a successful treatment.

There are many things to consider when figuring out what treatment is best. First, is a treatment needed at all? Some disorders go away with or without treatment just like the common cold, leaving nothing more than a bad memory. Others come and go but leave problems behind and still others come and stay.

Sometimes the best that can be done is to block or partially block your symptoms. Other times a cure can be found.

Sadly, insurance considerations can also dictate what treatment is offered. An HMO or other strictly managed health care insurance arrangement many times determines the treatment to be given and who will give it. Of course a person always has the option of looking for a treatment and paying out of their own pocket like we all used to do in the "old days."

A very ugly question may also have to be asked of a doctor: Is this the best possible treatment for me or for my insurance company? Don't assume a doctor will volunteer to give this information.

Treatment Talk

Doctors sometimes speak their own strange little language. The words may sound familiar but be careful, they may have a different meaning, a lot different than you might think.

When talking about treatment they may discuss control or improvement, rather than cure. Getting better or improving in doctor talk sometimes means that your situation will improve over what it is, not that the problem will disappear completely or that your life will go back to what it was. Significant improvement also doesn't mean cure, it means the improvement was enough to be meaningful or measurable to the doctor, not that a disease disappeared. If you want to know exactly how much improvement will occur, ask if you will get totally better or totally back to normal or words to that effect.

They may also refer to the side effects of a particular treatment as rare when the chance could be one in ten or one in twenty. That isn't rare to me and probably isn't to you either. If you can, get them to define their terms.

Always be specific in your descriptions and questions and don't assume you know what they mean or that they know what you mean during a discussion.

Over the next few chapters many different treatments will be covered including diet, medication, physical therapy, surgery and alternatives.

Next

Diet is covered in the next chapter.

Chapter Eleven
Diet

Diet changes can help a few vestibular disorders including allergies, migraine, and all types of endolymphatic hydrops including Meniere's Disease.

At best a diet change may reduce the number, frequency or severity of vertigo attacks and perhaps decrease the pressure and tinnitus. Diet isn't going to get rid of the underlying disease. There's also no way to predict ahead of time if a diet change will help at all. The only way to find out is through trial and error under a doctor's supervision.

Allergy

If a food allergy is known to be a problem simply not eating or drinking that food or anything containing it may help.

Some doctors recommend a food elimination diet when an allergy is suspected but the food unknown. An elimination diet is really used as a diagnostic test rather than a treatment. A symptom diary is kept while various foods are not eaten or eliminated from the diet. If symptoms improve or go away when a food has been stopped it's assumed the eliminated food was the problem and it's then avoided in the future.

In addition to the food elimination diet there's the rotating diet in which foods a person is allergic to are eaten only every 5 days or so.

Low Salt

Most doctors suggest a low salt diet, usually around 2500mg of sodium, for people with Meniere's disease or endolymphatic hydrops.

There are two theories for inner ear fluid problems:

- There's too much endolymph being produced by the inner ear
- The inner ear fluid regulating equipment is damaged and body wide shifts in fluid are felt in the ear

Doctors who feel too much endolymph is being produced prescribe a low-sodium diet. If the diet doesn't work after a few weeks a diet even lower in sodium might be suggested or a medication added or both.

In the case of the second theory the amount of sodium eaten must be decreased and evenly spread throughout the day. This means eating 6 little meals beginning first thing in the morning and ending an hour or two before bedtime.

Migraine
Food doesn't cause migraines to start up in the first place but a number of different foods are thought to bring on attacks in some people who suffer from migraines. Simply not eating those foods can help stop attacks. These foods include: Red wine, aged cheese (like cheddar), chocolate, citrus fruits and foods containing monosodium glutamate (MSG), nitrate or aspartame (artificial sweetener).

Carbohydrates
Doctors who feel general fluctuations in body fluids cause symptoms may also suggest limiting the simple carbohydrate foods and candies in the diet along with spreading out meals over the entire day.

Caffeine
Many doctors suggest eliminating caffeine from the diet. A low caffeine diet is thought, by the doctors recommending it, to improve circulation to the inner ear and within the inner ear.

Caffeine occurs naturally in chocolate (dark or semi-sweet has the most), coffee and tea (including green tea). It's added to a number of drinks such as Mountain Dew and is an ingredient in some over-the-counter anti-sleeping aids. Read all labels carefully when trying to avoid caffeine.

There's no way to predict ahead of time if a diet change will help. The only way to find out is through trial and error under a doctor's supervision. It can take weeks to see if a new diet's going to help.

Because a diet change has a very, very low chance of causing side effects it's a treatment that should be tried in both Meniere's disease and other cases of endolymphatic hydrops before going on to treatments with higher risk for problems.

Next
Medications are covered in the next chapter.

Chapter Twelve
Medications

In some cases medications can be used in the treatment of vestibular disorders. Before asking for, or taking, any medications a few things should be kept in mind. Most drugs, whether made by a pharmaceutical company or collected from the forest, are poisons and must be respected. None are 100% safe all of the time and all must be taken properly. They should only be used if you can commit to taking them correctly.

The medication descriptions and information appearing in this chapter are here to briefly introduce the drugs. The first and most important source of in-depth information about a drug should be the prescribing doctor and the pharmacist dispensing the drug. These professionals have information about interactions (when a drug acts differently when taken with other drugs or with food), how to take the drug (with food, without food) and any precautions that might be needed like avoiding alcohol or staying out of the sun.

Before taking a drug prescribed by a specialist it should be discussed with a PCP (Primary care provider), they're in the best position to know if the drug(s) can pose an overall health problem. People with diabetes mellitus, asthma, kidney disease, heart disease, liver disease, or glaucoma; those taking MAO inhibitors and women who might be pregnant or are breast-feeding must be particularly careful about this.

> **Note:** Drugs in this book appear in groups of drug families that are listed alphabetically, not in the order of importance.

Anti-Allergy

If the underlying problem causing the vestibular disorder is an allergy, or if an allergy increases the vestibular symptoms, anti-allergy or anti-inflammatory drugs might be useful. A doctor can prescribe allergy shots, anti-allergy drugs such as antihistamines and/or steroids.

> **Caution**: If using betahistine HCl, also known as Serc, don't use any antihistamines without discussing it with the prescribing doctor. The two sets of drugs could cancel each other out.

It's not unusual for anti-allergy drugs to cause some drowsiness and loss of coordination.

Don't drive or operate dangerous machinery (power tools, lawn mower, ladders) or do anything else that requires balance and/or coordination etc. while taking these drugs.

Antibiotic

Antibiotics are not a common treatment for inner ear problems since bacteria cause very few. The two disorders that should be treated with antibiotics are otosyphilis and bacterial labyrinthitis.

If sinusitis or middle ear infections are creating or worsening vestibular symptoms, treatment with antibiotics might help.

One antibiotic, gentamicin, is given at times as a treatment to destroy vestibular function. There's more about this later in the chapter.

Anti-Immune System

In some situations the body is attacked by it's own immune system. This is called an autoimmune reaction or disease. Many of these diseases are the rheumatologist's particular area of the medical world, not an otologist or neurotologist. To help with both the diagnosis and treatment when an autoimmune reaction is suspected most otologists and neurotologists send their patients to a rheumatologist.

> **Note:** The American College of Rheumatology describes a rheumatologist as "an internist or pediatrician who is qualified by additional training and experience in the diagnosis and treatment of arthritis and other diseases of the joints, muscles and bones. Rheumatologists treat arthritis, certain autoimmune diseases, musculoskeletal pain disorders and osteoporosis. There are more than 100 types of these diseases, including rheumatoid arthritis, osteoarthritis, gout, lupus, back pain, osteoporosis, fibromyalgia and tendonitis."

Stopping the immune system in its tracks requires drugs that are real heavyweights. They not only stop the immune system from attacking the body, they also keep it from doing the work it's supposed to do, i.e. protecting a person from infection. Treatment should not be started unless you are willing to take the drugs exactly as prescribed and participate in the treatment by actively watching for problems.

When following the instructions of the rheumatologist, neurotologist, PCP and pharmacist the drugs can be taken in relative safety. When taken improperly or without watching carefully, serious problems can occur.

It's very important to be on the lookout for infections when taking anti-immune system drugs. Body temperature should be checked every day at the same time. New or increased fatigue, sore throat, runny nose, red or swollen areas or burning when urinating should be reported to a doctor. Abnormal bleeding can also occur. Report any nosebleeds, bleeding gums, bruising or black looking stools. Other changes to report include very dark urine, yellowing of the skin, yellowing of the whites of the eyes, clay colored stools and general itching.

Steroids

The oldest and best-known anti-immune system drugs (also called immune suppressors) are the steroids. Not only are they able to calm down the immune system they can also reduce inflammation. Two of the steroids in common use are Prednisone and Decadron (dexamethasone).

At times steroids can also be used to help make the diagnosis of an autoimmune disorder. If there's an improvement while using them an autoimmune diagnosis can be considered and if they don't help it might be ruled out. Steroids may be continued after the diagnosis of an immune problem is made or might be replaced by another drug with fewer side effects.

Although steroids are a natural body chemical, many serious side effects can occur when they are given by pill or injection over weeks, months or years. These drugs must be viewed as potential trouble- makers and not as harmless, natural substances. Let your PCP know if another doctor prescribes these for you. The number of side effects a person experiences from these usually depends upon the amount of the drug taken and the length of time it's been taken. The higher the dose and longer it's taken the greater the number of side effects and the more serious they may be.

Caution: If you remember nothing else about steroids it's this: ***DO NOT STOP TAKING THEM SUDDENLY OR ON YOUR OWN***—there can be he—to pay if you do.

When taking extra steroids the body stops making the natural ones and comes to rely totally on the pills or injections. If the pills are stopped suddenly there won't be enough steroids in the body to carry out normal functions and extreme problems can begin.

Wear a medic alert bracelet to let health care professionals know steroids are being taken. The Medic Alert Foundation can be found online at www.medicalert.org or written to at 2323 Colorado Ave., Turlock, CA 95382.

When having dental work done let the dentist know you are on steroids. Steroids may not be the right treatment for people with diabetes mellitus, history of chronic infections, tuberculosis, high blood pressure, active herpes simplex, myasthenia gravis, thrombophlebitis, hypothyroidism or if HIV positive.

There just isn't enough room in this book to fit all the important things people on high doses or long-term use of steroids should know. Anyone who will be on them for months or longer should get more information from his or her doctor and pharmacist.

The most common side effects during short-term use are sleeplessness, mood swings, weight gain and fluid retention. Stomach upset is also relatively common.

Methotrexate (Rhematrex)
This drug began its life as an anti-cancer drug, but is now widely used at a lower dose to combat psoriasis, rheumatoid arthritis and now, inner ear autoimmune disorders. It's comes as a pill, is taken weekly and can take as long as 6 to 12 weeks to start working. It should NOT be taken with food. Blood work is done occasionally to check the blood count, uric acid level, kidney function and liver function. Lung (pulmonary) function testing and/or chest X-Rays may also be done.

People with stomach ulcer, kidney disease, anemia, liver disease, or alcoholism: woman who are nursing or pregnant, and those who are HIV positive may be excluded from taking this drug.

A rash, redness or mouth sores appearing while on this drug should be reported to the prescribing doctor.

Enbrel (Etanercept)
This new drug was developed and marketed for use in rheumatoid arthritis but some doctors are now using it for autoimmune inner ear disorders too. In addition to stopping the immune system it also reduces inflammation.

Technical point: Enbrel is an anti-tumor necrosis factor drug. Tumor necrosis factor (TNF) is a cytokine involved in inflammatory and immune responses.

People with chicken pox, a history of chronic infections, are HIV positive or women who are pregnant or breast-feeding may be excluded from using the drug. While undergoing treatment with Enbrel a person should not be vaccinated with a live vaccine such as the small pox vaccine or inhaled Flu vaccine. More information is available at www.enbrel.com

One potential drawback is that Enbrel is given by injection, not by pill.

Anti-Migraine

Medications are used in two ways for migraines, to prevent the migraine or to stop it while in progress.

Migraine prevention drugs include beta-blockers (Propranolol), calcium channel blockers (Verapamil), tricyclics (amitriptyline), serotonin re-uptake inhibitors (Prozac), non-steroidal anti-inflammatories (Naproxen), clonidine and depakote.

The drugs in most widespread use to stop or abort a migraine are the triptans such as imitrex.

In addition, woman may be helped by taking female hormones if the migraines are occurring during certain times of their menstrual cycle.

Anti-Virals

If a disorder might be caused by a virus an antiviral drug may be prescribed. Famciclovir (Famvir), acyclovir (Zovirax) and Valacyclovir (Vatrex) are three of the anti-virals effective against the herpes simplex virus (HSV-1 and HSV-2) and herpes zoster.

They work by preventing the virus cell from making DNA. These are most effective for herpes zoster (shingles) when started within the first 48 hours of the infection.

These drugs are routinely used for ear shingles and may also be used in other situations such as vestibular neuronitis or labyrinthitis as well.

When acyclovir is used for a period of time blood work should be done to check the blood count and kidney function.

Calcium Channel Blockers

Calcium channel blockers are drugs that change the way calcium enters a body cell through calcium channels. This may work right in the vestibular hair cells since these have calcium channels.

Two calcium channel blockers, cinnarizine and flunarizine, are commonly used in Europe for motion sickness and Meniere's disease. In addition to their calcium channel blocking abilities these drugs are also antihistamines, H-1 antihistamines. Cinnarizine and flunarizine aren't approved by the Food and Drug Administration for use in the U.S. However, some U.S. doctors prescribe the calcium channel blocker verapamil that is available here.

Verapamil isn't for everyone. Its major use in health care is to treat high blood pressure, angina and/or irregular heartbeats. People with heart problems, including irregular heartbeat, arrhythmia, may be excluded from using it for migraines. The drug should not be stopped suddenly and people taking it should stay well hydrated and eat lots of fiber. The prescribing doctor should be called if swelling occurs.

Diuretics

In addition to diet changes, folks with Meniere's disease, and other forms of endolymphatic hydrops, may also be prescribed a diuretic. The idea is to stabilize the inner ear fluid balance or reduce the amount of fluid in the inner ear. It's important to understand that diuretics are aimed at the increase in the amount of endolymph caused by the disease and won't make the disease itself go away.

A diuretic reduces the amount of fluids in the body by forcing the kidneys to get rid of sodium (Na+). An important side effect of diuretics is their affect on potassium (K+). Some do nothing to potassium, others reduce the amount in the blood stream and some actually increase the potassium level. Diuretics are either potassium wasting or potassium sparing. With wasting diuretics, potassium is lost from the body and may need to be replaced. In sparing diuretics, potassium is kept in the body and may rise to abnormally high levels. A potassium problem can only be accurately diagnosed with a simple, inexpensive blood test. How a diuretic will behave in a particular person can't always be predicted.

In a perfect world blood tests would be done before starting a diuretic and then in a week or two after starting to use it. In a not so perfect world it will be checked a few weeks after starting the drug. If your neurotologist doesn't order any blood work at all go through your PCP to get it done.

Don't dehydrate yourself while taking a diuretic unless your doctor has specifically told you to do so and even then discuss it with your PCP. The body needs both water and salt (sodium) to work properly.

There are many diuretics around. The one most commonly used in the U.S. for inner ear problems is hydrochlorothiazide (HCTZ) either plain or in combination with another drug, triamterene. HCTZ and triamterene is the combination found in the prescription drugs Dyazide, Maxzide and Maxzide-25.

Acetazolamide (Diamox), furosemide (Lasix), methazolamide (Neptazone) and spironolactone (Aldactone) are other diuretics in use.

There are differences between the many diuretics, so if one doesn't work, another might.

Gentamicin

Gentamicin is a member of the aminoglycoside antibiotic family. The first aminoglycoside, streptomycin, was developed in the mid-1940's to treat tuberculosis, the deadliest infectious disease of that time. Soon after the drug went on the market it was discovered streptomycin could cause inner ear poisoning (ototoxicity) resulting in vestibular symptoms, hearing loss and balance function impairment in some people.

It didn't take ENT's long to figure out they might be able to use this vestibular poisoning to the advantage of people with Meniere's disease having uncontrollable attacks of violent vertigo. Instead of doing surgery to destroy the inner ear they figured the damaged areas could be destroyed chemically, a procedure sometimes referred to as a chemical labyrinthectomy.

Streptomycin was the first drug used to intentionally destroy inner ear balance function. The drug was injected into a large muscle from where it entered the blood stream and poisoned both ears. Attempts to poison one ear were less successful because injecting streptomycin directly into an ear caused massive loss of hearing. Gentamicin was developed in the 1960's and has become a popular treatment in part because it doesn't cause the same degree of hearing loss. Gentamicin treatments seem to work best in stopping spontaneous attacks of violent vertigo, usually from Meniere's disease. Vertigo and nausea from head movement or vision aren't usually helped by it unless spontaneous attacks of violent vertigo are occurring along with them.

Because its effects are destructive and permanent gentamicin should not be rushed into or used as a first treatment. Other less harmful treatments such as diuretics and diet change or betahistine should be tried first.

Gentamicin is placed into the middle ear from where it can diffuse into the inner ear. There are several ways this can be done:

- Injection of gentamicin through the ear drum with a small syringe in an office procedure (this causes a burning sensation for a minute or two in some people)

- Minor office surgery in which a tube is inserted through the ear drum, a wick placed through that and ear drops placed into the ear canal at home as directed by a doctor
- Operating room procedure in which a tube is inserted through the eardrum, a catheter passed through the tube until one end is against the round window and the other end attached to a small pump that continuously sends gentamicin into the ear for days to weeks
- In a method that isn't used very often gentamicin crystals can be placed against the round window in a one-time operating room procedure

These four methods are referred to as either transtympanic or intratympanic administration of gentamicin.

All the procedures carry some risk with them. The eardrum hole may not close on it's own, an infection could occur, hearing might be lost and permanent balance impairment could occur.

Gentamicin treatment aims to stop the spontaneous attacks of violent vertigo by killing off the bad vestibular hair cells and may also decrease the amount of endolymph made by the inner ear.

The idea, when possible, is to kill off just enough bad vestibular hair cells to stop the spontaneous attacks of violent vertigo. The term chemical labyrinthectomy isn't accurate because the aim isn't complete destruction and, unlike a surgical labyrinthectomy hearing isn't sacrificed, at least not intentionally.

Gentamicin therapy is done a bit by trial and error because each person and their ear are so very different. One standard amount isn't going to work for every person. Doses must be determined on a case-by-case basis with each person watched very carefully to determine when enough has been given. Hearing, balance and the VOR (vestibulocular reflex) should be tested before, during and after the treatment and injections stopped if hearing loss occurs. VEMP testing can also be done to check on vestibular function. The drug might also be stopped if too much balance impairment occurs.

In a number of people the vertigo returns and another round of gentamicin is needed. Why? Some of the "bad" hair cells may have only been damaged and are able to heal up and come back to life. Gentamicin also doesn't stop the Meniere's disease from progressing so it can spread to other hair cells that may still be alive. Symptoms can start up again if those hair cells weren't killed by the gentamicin.

Hearing loss is possible from the use of gentamicin. In general the larger the dose of gentamicin the higher the risk of hearing loss and the closer together the doses are given the greater the risk to hearing. In other words if gentamicin is given in one big dose once or twice a day everyday for several days the chance of a hearing loss is very high compared to one low dose every two weeks or more. Procedures using a pump to deliver the drug also appear to have a lesser chance of causing hearing loss.

Caution: This treatment causes a permanent loss of at least some vestibular function that may or may not be a problem now or in the future. The treatment cannot be reversed and some people do end up in a worse situation than they started out in.

The symptoms of vestibular destruction range from nothing to strong vertigo and vomiting for days. What a person will experience depends upon:

- How much vestibular function is left in the ear when the treatment is begun
- The amount of destruction done by the treatment

- How rapidly the damage occurs

The strongest symptoms come from rapid, massive damage in an ear that had lots of good vestibular hair cells left.

After treatment with gentamicin some people hardly miss a day of work while others feel ill and need vestibular rehabilitation to get back to full speed. It's unknown what percentage of people receiving gentamicin has a change in their ear fullness and/or tinnitus.

Histamines

Histamine is a chemical made throughout the body and brain. It does many things such as increasing the amount of stomach acids, tightening lung muscles and increasing the size of the smallest blood vessels in the body. The redness seen after a mosquito bite and around injured areas as well as the redness and swelling of allergies are all from histamine.

A few doctors give histamine to people with Meniere's disease in the hope it will increase the blood supply to the inner ear and reduce symptoms. It's given as a drop in the mouth or intravenously.

When histamine is given to people with allergies, asthma, low blood pressure, pheochromocytoma, peptic ulcer or too much stomach acid it can cause problems. If an antihistamine is given to someone undergoing treatment with histamine the drugs may cancel each other out.

> **Special note:** If you are having allergy testing, tell the allergist that you have received histamine or betahistine and when you had the last dose.

Betahistine (Serc)

Betahistine is very similar to histamine and is considered a histamine analog. That means it isn't chemically identical to histamine but resembles it so closely it can act like it. This drug is widely used for Meniere's disease throughout the world—with the exception of the U.S.

> **Technical point:** More formally called betahistine dihydrochloride.

Serc was studied in the U.S., received FDA approval and made available in 1966 but was removed from the market in 1972 after the original studies were determined to contain "deficiencies" and "misrepresentations."

That isn't the end of the story for this drug in the U.S. A doctor, or other health care professional authorized to write prescriptions, can still legally prescribe it and the drug can be filled outside the U.S. or prepared in a U.S. pharmacy equipped to do drug compounding.

> **Note:** Compounding is the preparation of a drug from raw products or ingredients. All pharmacists are trained during their schooling to compound drugs, but most don't routinely provide the service in their pharmacies.

There is some research evidence suggesting Serc can improve the symptoms of Meniere's disease and may do so through an effect on the circulation in the inner ear. The manufacturer recommends 16mg 3 times a day but some doctors and patients have found that a higher dose is required to stop the attacks of Meniere's disease.

The use of betahistine in people with asthma, peptic ulcer or stomach acid overproduction, pheochromocytoma and during pregnancy or breastfeeding isn't highly recommended.

Betahistine's action may also be reduced or prevented by the use of antihistamines at the same time. Reported side effects include gastrointestinal disturbances, headache and skin rashes.

Steroids Into the Ear

Steroids can also be injected into the ear in a procedure called transtympanic or intratympanic steroid injection. Most doctors use the steroid dexamethasone (Decadron) for the procedure. It's placed into the middle ear from where it diffuses into the inner ear.

The steroid can be placed into the ear in a number of ways:

- Syringe injection through the eardrum right in the doctors office
- Dropped into the ear canal from where it passes through a surgically implanted tube (done with a simple office procedure) into the middle ear
- Dripped in via micropump after surgically implanting a catheter in the operating room

This treatment does carry the risk of middle ear infection and failure of the eardrum hole (perforation) to heal. (Some will heal on their own while others require surgery to close up.)

Symptom Blockers

Some drugs can't stop the vestibular disease or reverse damage that's been done, but they can block symptoms, at least to some degree. If they cover up vestibular symptoms they're called vestibular suppressants and if they reduce nausea and vomiting they're called antiemetics.

This section contains only a sample of the drugs available in the U.S. Symptom blockers are NOT a good treatment when used instead of finding and treating the actual cause of a vestibular disorder. They're also a bad choice for a disorder that causes only loss of vestibular function such as ototoxicity. However, when the cause can't be found, or there is no treatment, they can be a real lifesaver in people with strong symptoms from a fluctuating vestibular disorder. When given for the right reasons they can be a terrific help. People do feel a lot better when there's no vertigo.

Symptom blockers do have some drawbacks:

- Vestibular tests are messed up by taking vestibular suppressants and/or antiemetics
- They can probably interfere with the normal way the body adapts to the loss of vestibular function
- The drowsiness they cause can make driving and operating machinery and power tools dangerous (don't climb ladders or so anything else requiring good balance and coordination while under the effect of these drugs)
- In exchange for less vestibular symptoms, balance function may worsen
- They can cause drowsiness and blurred vision and make a person feel quite a bit worse (which may be mistaken for worsening of the vestibular problem)
- Alcohol must be avoided when taking many of these drugs
- Memory and thought can be interfered with at times
- Meclizine, cyclizine, dimenhydrinate and promethazine can interfere with allergy testing

Some vestibular suppressants, like meclizine and dimenhydrinate, can be purchased over-the-counter, others must be prescribed. Many drugs from a number of drug classes are available.

Anti-Motion Sickness/Anti-Nausea/Vomiting
Ginger
This food substance is well known to help decrease the nausea and vomiting of motion sickness, pregnancy and surgery, in some people. It's a food that can be eaten in many ways such as ginger ale, ginger snap cookies, pickled ginger or as a capsule that can be purchased in the vitamin and supplements section of most drug stores and grocery stores.

Ginger works in the stomach rather than in the brain so there's no drowsiness, or any other disturbing side effects from the drug.

Dimenhydrinate (Dramamine Original)
Dimenhydrinate is used by many people to prevent motion sickness and nausea/vomiting and may also be prescribed for vestibular symptoms. It's an antihistamine of the H-1 type and available as a pill. This drug is marketed as Dramamine Original and might be easily confused with Dramamine Less Drowsy, an entirely different drug.

Meclizine (Antivert, Dramamine less drowsy)
Meclizine is an antihistamine type drug widely used to prevent motion sickness and nausea. It's also sometimes prescribed for vestibular symptoms and nausea/vomiting. This drug is also an antihistamine of the H-1 type and available as a pill.

Meclizine is marketed by one company under the name Dramamine Less Drowsy and might be confused with Dramamine Original, an entirely different drug.

Promethazine (Phenergan)
Promethazine is a phenothiazine derivative. It has an advantage over dimenhydrinate and meclizine, because in addition to being made in pill form it also comes as a suppository which can't be vomited back up. This drug helps a lot of people with their nausea and vomiting but its success with vertigo is hit or miss. This may be because the drug is most effective in preventing motion sickness, not in treating it once it has begun.

It should NOT be taken daily for months or years on end because it can cause a permanent side effect called an extrapyramidal reaction consisting of any of a number of involuntary movement problems. These symptoms can also be produced by prochlorperazine, also known as Stemetil in English speaking countries outside the U.S.

Extrapyramidal reactions/disorders include:

- Akathisia—The inability to sit still
- Tardive dyskinesia—Involuntary face and tongue movement that may be constant
- Athetosis—Constant, slow, involuntary movement of the fingers, toes, hands and feet in which they are placed palm up and then palm down
- Hemiballism—Involuntary movement of the arm and leg on one side of the body that looks like jerking

Scopolamine (transdermal scopolamine)
Scopolamine is an anti-cholinergic and belladonna alkaloid drug delivered through the skin from a patch applied behind the ear. The drug affect begins a couple of hours after being applied and continues up to 72 hours.

Transdermal scopolamine is not meant for constant, long-term use because it's addictive and on rare occasion hospitalization for detoxification is necessary when stopping the drug.

Anti-nausea.Anti-vomiting

Caution: All of the drugs in this class are capable of causing the above-mentioned extrapyramidal symptoms and should not be taken regularly for long periods of time.

Ondansetron (Zofran)

Ondansetron is approved for the nausea and vomiting of chemotherapy and radiation therapy and is used on occasion for the nausea and vomiting of vestibular disorders. It's a member of the newer selective serotonin 5-HT3 receptor antagonist drug group that blocks the action of serotonin. It stops vomiting signals that are made by the release of serotonin.

Ondansetron is an expensive drug but may help if other, cheaper, drugs aren't working.

Caution: Asparatame enters the system when taking this drug.

Prochlorperazine (Compazine, Stemetil)

Prochlorperzaine is used for nausea and vomiting in the U.S. In the United Kingdom it's also used as a vestibular suppressor.

This drug works in the brain to stop nausea and vomiting from any cause. It has many more side effects than drugs such as meclizine (see above) and can cause extrapyramidal reactions. In addition to being manufactured in pill form it's also available as a suppository so it can be taken even when vomiting.

Benzodiazepines (Valium, etc.)

Drugs of the benzodiazepine family, including Valium, Klonopin, and Xanax, may be prescribed to help block abnormal movement sensations such as vertigo. These drugs help some people almost dramatically and others not at all. These drugs can also reduce muscle tension, anxiety and seizure activity. Xanax also reduces tinnitus in some people.

They are thought to work in the brain and might do so by an action on GABA, one of the neurotransmitters in the brain.

Their major drawback is addiction. There's a 50% chance of having withdrawal symptoms when the drug is stopped after 8 months or more of use although they can also be seen when the drug has been used as little as 4 to 6 weeks. Benzodiazepines can also lead to depression and trouble thinking.

DO NOT suddenly stop taking these drugs if they have been taken daily for more than 4 to 6 weeks. Most drug experts feel the way to stop taking them is to decrease the original amount by about 25% each week.

Stopping or reducing the dosage of benzodiazepines can lead to the following situations in some people:

- Withdrawal—The start of new symptoms as a result of stopping a drug
- Relapse—A gradual return of the original symptoms
- Rebound—A return of the original symptoms at a more intense level

Miscellaneous
Gabapentin (Neurontin)
Gabapentin is an anti-seizure drug used very occasionally to suppress vestibular symptoms. It's chemical formula looks very similar to GABA, a brain chemical neurotransmitter, but how it works is unknown. Blood counts should be done if taking this drug long-term.

Serotonin manipulating drugs
Drugs of both the tricyclic antidepressant family and the SSRI's (selective serotonin reuptake inhibitors) are used for their antidepressant action and lessen vestibular symptoms in some people.

The tricyclics include: amitriptyline (Elavil), imipramine (Tofranil), nortriptyline (Pamelor) and desipramine (Norpramine). The SSRI's include Prozac (fluoxetine), Zoloft (sertraline), Paxil (paroxetine), Luvox (fluvoxamine) and Celexa (citalopram).

How they work is unknown but most theories revolve around an affect on neurotransmitters, the chemicals that carry on the work of the nervous system.

Some adults are supersensitive to their effects and may need a very small dose such as the amount a young child might take. Both fluoxetine and paroxetin are available in liquid form that allows the smallest doses.

Stopping these drugs suddenly can lead to rebound symptoms, a return of the prior symptoms at a much higher level. A few people also experience trouble with balance and may develop new vestibular symptoms when suddenly stopping the drugs.

Getting More Drug Information
Start with your doctor and pharmacist when you need more information about drugs. If they aren't giving you enough information you have three options, stop searching for more information, change to a doctor who will give you the information you want or do your own work.

Sum Up
Many drugs are available for vestibular disorders and the symptoms they cause.

Next
Physical therapy will be covered in the next chapter.

References and Reading List:
Baylla, B.W. "Update on intratympanic gentamicin for Meniere's disease." *Laryngoscope, 110*(2 Pt 1):236-240, 2000.

Brookes, G.B. "Meniere's Disease: A practical approach to management." *Drugs*, 25:77-89, 1983.

Dziadziola, J.K., Laurikainen, E.L., Rachel, J.D., and Quirk, W.S. "Betahistine increases vestibular blood flow." *Otolaryngology-Head and Neck Surgery, 120*(3):400-405, 1999.

Eklund, S., Pyykko, I., Aalto, H., Ishizaki, H., and Vasama, J.P. "Effect of intratympanic gentamicin on hearing and tinnitus in Meniere's disease." *American Journal of Otology*, 20(3):350-356, 1999.

Ell, J., and Gresty, M. "The effects of the "vestibular sedative" drug Flunarizine upon the vestibular and oculomotor systems." *Journal of Neurology, Neurosurgery and Psychology*, 45:716-724, 1983.

Forge, A., and Schnacht, J. "Aminoglycoside antibiotics." *Audiology and Neurotology*, 5:3-22, 2000.

Gorman, J.M. *Essential guide to psychiatric drugs.* Third edition. New York: St. Martin's Press, 1997.

Graham, M. "Bilateral Meniere's disease: Treatment with intramuscular titration streptomycin sulfate." *Otolaryngologic Clinics of North America*, *30*(6):1097-1100, 1997.

Haid, T. "Evaluation of flunarizine in patients with Meniere's disease: subjective and vestibular findings." *Acta Otolaryngologica*, Supplement *460*:149-153, 1988.

Hardman, G., and Limbird, J. *Goodman and Gilman's the pharmacological basis of therapeutics.* Tenth edition. New York: McGraw-Hill Professional, 2001.

Harner, S.G., Driscoll, C.L., Facer, G.W., Beatty, C.W., and McDonald, T.J. "Long-term follow-up of transtympanic gentamicin for Meniere's syndrome." *Otology and Neurotology*, *22*(2):210-214, 2001.

Hellstrom, S., and Odkvist, L. "Pharmacologic labyrinthectomy." *Otolaryngologic Clinics of North America*, *27*(2):307-315, 1994.

Hirsch, B.E., and Kamerer, D.B. "Role of chemical labyrinthectomy in the treatment of Meniere's disease." *Otolaryngologic Clinics of North America, 30(6):1039-1049, 1997.*

Hoffer, M.E., Kopke, R.D., Weisskopf, P., Gottshall, K., Allen, K., Wester, D., and Balaban C. "Use of the round window microcatheter in the treatment of Meniere's disease." *Laryngoscope, 111*:2046-2049, 2001.

Hone, S.W., Nedzelski, J., and Chen, J. "Does intratympanic gentamicin treatment for Meniere's disease cause complete vestibular ablation?" *Journal of Otolaryngology*, *29*(2):83-87, 2000.

Itoh, A., and Sakata, E. "Treatment of vestibular disorders." *Acta Otolaryngologica*, Supplement 481:617-623, 1991.

Kaplan, D.M., Nedzelski, J.M., Al-Abidi, A., Chen, J.M., and Shipp, D.B. "Hearing loss following intratympanic instillation of gentamicin for the treatment of unilateral Meniere's disease." *Journal of Otolaryngology*, *31*(2):106-111, 2002.

Kingma, H., Bonink M., Meulenbroeks, A., and Konijnenberg, H. "Dose-dependent effect of betahistine on the vestibulo-ocular reflex: a double-blind placebo controlled study in patients with paroxysmal vertigo." *Acta Otolaryngologica, 117*(5):641-646, 1997.

King, W.P. "The use of low-dose histamine therapy in otolaryngology." *Ear Nose Throat Journal*, 79:366-368, 1999.

Lacour, M., and Sterkers, O. "Histamine and betahistine in the treatment of vertigo: elucidation of mechanisms of action." *CNS Drugs, 15*(11):853-870, 2001.

Langner, E., Greifenberg, S., and Gruenwald, J. "Ginger: History and use." *Advances in Therapy, 15(1):25-44, 1998.*

LaRouere, M.J., Zappia, J.J., and Graham, M.D. "Titration streptomycin therapy in Meniere's disease: current Concepts." *American Journal of Otology, 14*(5):474-477, 1993.

Lassen, L.F., Hirsch, B.E., and Kamerer, D.B. "Use of nimodipine in the medical treatment of Meniere's disease: clinical experience." *American Journal of Otology, 17*(4):577-580, 1996.

Laurikainen, E., Miller, J.F., and Pyykko, I. "Betahistine effects on cochlear blood flow: from the laboratory to the clinic." *Acta Otolaryngologica,* Supplement 544:5-7, 2000.

Leutje, C.M., and Wooten, J. "Clinical manifestations of transdermal scopolamine addiction." *Ear Nose Throat Journal,* 75(4):210-214, 1996.

Longridge, N.S., and Mallinson, A.I. "Low-dose intratympanic gentamicin treatment for dizziness in Meniere's disease." *Journal of Otolaryngology, 29*(1):35-39, 2000.

Marzo, S.J., and Leonetti, J.P. "Intratympanic gentamicin therapy for persistent vertigo after endolymphatic sac surgery." *Otolaryngology-Head and Neck Surgery, 126*(1):31-33, 2002.

Mira, E. "Betahistine in the treatment of vertigo. History and clinical implications of recent pharmacological researches." *Acta Otorhinolaryngologica Italiano, 21*(3 Supplement 66):1-7, 2001.

Monsell, E.M., Cass, S.P., and Ryback, L.P. "Therapeutic use of aminoglycosides in Meniere's disease." *Otolaryngologic Clinics of North America, 26*(5):737-746, 1993.

Nadel, D.M. "The use of systemic steroids in otolaryngology." *Ear Nose and Throat Journal, 75:*502-516, 1996.

Norris, C.H. "Drugs affecting the inner ear: a review of their clinical efficacy, mechanisms of action, toxicity, and place in therapy." *Drugs, 36:*754-772, 1988.

Perry, P.J., Alexander, B., and Liskow, B. *Psychotropic drug handbook.* Seventh edition. Washington, D.C.: American Psychiatric Press, 1997.

Rascol, O., Hain, T.C., Brefell, C., Benazet, M., Claret, M., and Montastruc, J.L. "Antivertigo medications and drug-induced vertigo. A pharmacological review." *Drugs,* 50(5):777-791, 1995.

Ruckenstein, M.J., Rutka, J.A., and Hawke, M. "The Treatment of Meniere's Disease: Torok Revisited." *Laryngoscope, 101:*211-218, 1991.

Santos, P.M., Hall, R.A., Snyder, J.M., Hughes, L.F., and Dobie, R.A. "Diuretic and diet effect on Meniere's disease evaluated by the 1985 Committee on Hearing and Equilibrium Guidelines." *Otolaryngology-Head and Neck Surgery, 109*(4):680-689, 1993.

Scherer, J.C., and Roach, S.S. *Introductory clinical pharmacology.* Fifth edition. Philadelphia: Lippincott, 1996.

Schoendorf, J., Neugebauer, P., and Michel, O. "Continuous intratympanic infusion of gentamicin via a microcatheter in Meniere's disease." *Otolaryngology-Head and Neck Surgery, 124*(2):203-207, 2001.

Sennaroglu, L., Sennaroglu, G., Gursel, B., and Dini, F.M. "Intratympanic dexamethasone, intratympanic gentamicin, and endolymphatic sac surgery for intractable vertigo in Meniere's disease." *Otolaryngology-Head and Neck Surgery, 125*(5):537-543, 2001.

Shea, J.J., and Ge, X. "Dexamethasone perfusion of the labyrinth plus intravenous dexamethasone for Meniere's disease." *Otolaryngologic Clinics of North America, 29*(2):353-358, 1996.

Shea, J.J. "The role of dexamethasone or streptomycin perfusion in the treatment of Meniere's Disease." *Otolaryngologic Clinics of North America, 30*(6):1051-1059, 1997.

Silverman, H.M. *The pill book.* Seventh edition. New York: Bantam Books, 1996.

Silverstein, H., Arruda, J., Rosenberg, S.I., Deems, D., and Hester, T.O. "Direct round window membrane application of gentamicin in the treatment of Meniere's disease." *Otolaryngology-Head and Neck Surgery, 120*(5):649-655, 1999.

Silverstein, H., Choo, D., Rosenberg, S.I., Kuhn, J., Seidman, M., and Stein, I. "Intratympanic Steroid Treatment of Inner Ear Disease and Tinnitus (Preliminary Report)." *Ear Nose and Throat Journal, 75*(8):4468-4474, 1996.

Slattery, W.H., and Fayad, J.N. "Medical treatment of Meniere's disease." *Otolaryngologic Clinics of North America, 3*(6):1027-1037, 1997.

Staab, J.P. "Diagnosis and treatment of psychologic symptoms and psychiatric disorders in patients with dizziness and imbalance." *Otolaryngologic Clinics of North America,* 33(3):617-635, 2000.

Staab, J.P., Ruckenstein, M.J., Solomon, D., and Shepard, N.T. "Serotonin reuptake inhibitors for dizziness with psychiatric symptoms." *Archives of Otolaryngology-Head and Neck Surgery,* 128:554-560, 2002.

Verspeelt, J., De Locht, P., and Amery, W.K. "Postmarketing study of the use of flunarizine in vestibular vertigo and in migraine." *European Journal of Clinical Pharmacology, 51*(1):15-22, 1996.

Walsted, A. "Unpredictable hearing loss after intratympanic gentamicin treatment for vertigo. A new theory." *Acta Otolaryngologica, 121*(1):42-44, 2001.

Wanamaker, H.H., Slepecky, N.B., Cefaratti, L.K., and Ogata, Y. "Comparison of vestibular and cochlear ototoxicity from transtympanic streptomycin administration." *American Journal of Otology, 20*(4):457-464, 1999.

Chapter Thirteen
Physical Therapy

Vestibular rehabilitation therapy (VRT) or physical therapy for vestibular disorders is an exercise treatment for both the symptoms and poor balance of vestibular disorders. The exercises usually involve eye movement, head movement, body movement, standing and walking. They won't get rid of the underlying cause of the disorder but can improve balance and possibly stop or improve the symptoms of a disorder.

Right now this treatment is in a bit of a confused state in the U.S. It's only been in general use since the 1990's and some of the health care professionals performing it haven't received much more than a weekend course to guide them, some have no formal education in this specialty at all. There is no professional organization offering a certification program and within health care it's unclear who should be providing the service. On one end vestibular rehabilitation therapy is done by an experienced, state-licensed physical therapist with a masters degree while on the other hand it's done by anyone a doctor assigns to the job.

Who Can Be Helped?
People with a wide range of disorders have been helped to better balance and/or improvement of symptoms with VRT.

Unfortunately there's one general category of disorders that can't be helped as much as the others, those that cause function to fluctuate frequently like Meniere's disease. If attacks of violent vertigo occur more frequently than every 3 to 4 weeks most experts feel vestibular rehabilitation therapy is less helpful because every time an attack comes on it knocks a person back to square one.

The only way to find out if vestibular rehabilitation therapy will help is to give it a good try for several weeks or months.

How Is It Done?
VRT begins with a history and examination to determine general physical condition, balance ability, muscle strength, joint flexibility, symptoms, actions that bring symptoms on, and how much you rely on vision, proprioception and vestibular information for balance.

A computerized machine may also be used to look at balance ability. After the therapist is done with all this they determine what's needed, set a goal and give instructions and demonstrations for exercises to be done at home. The exercise program is based on the history, examination and symptoms, not on the diagnosis (except in benign paroxysmal positional vertigo). Reassessments are done every week or two and changes made as needed.

Unfortunately the vestibular rehabilitation therapy exercises make some people feel more off balance and nauseated for the first few days of therapy and sometimes each time new exercises are added. When undergoing vestibular rehabilitation therapy keep in mind the saying, no pain, no gain. There's no pain to these exercises but there can be a little bit of suffering that must be toughed out for short periods of time. They should not bring on ear fullness or pain, tinnitus and/or hearing loss. If any of these appear therapy should be stopped immediately and the doctor who ordered the VRT notified.

People who work outside the home may want to start the exercises and make changes in them on Friday evenings so they have the weekend to recuperate from any ill effects.

Taking symptom reducing drugs like meclizine or Valium or drinking alcohol probably reduces the effectiveness of the exercises. If you need any of these drugs talk to your therapist about how to proceed.

The Goals of VRT:

- Assist the brain's normal adjustment to a vestibular loss
- Force the brain to adjust to a vestibular loss
- Increase reliance on vestibular information
- Become accustomed to bad vestibular information
- Increase reliance on vision and proprioception
- Improve the vestibulocular reflex
- Increase muscle strength
- Increase joint flexibility
- Gain balance practice and experience

Each person will have different needs requiring different goals. For example: One person might need to increase their use of vision and another might need to decrease it.

Assisting the brain's normal adjustment to a partial vestibular loss
When a partial loss of vestibular function occurs, the brain immediately begins the natural process of vestibular compensation. Therapy can be aimed at helping this along a bit by encouraging the use of vision and movement, two activities crucial for vestibular compensation.

A partial loss includes any of the following situations:

- Reduced information from one ear
- Reduced information from both ears
- No information at all from one ear
- No information at all from one ear and reduced information from the other

The term vestibular compensation refers specifically to the chemical changes that occur in the brain allowing it to continue carrying out its balance function after a partial vestibular loss. The adjustment to total loss in each ear requires a different process called sensory substitution.

Forcing the brain to adjust to a vestibular loss
Sometimes after a partial loss of vestibular function the brain doesn't automatically or thoroughly undergo vestibular compensation. In this case a rigorous program of vision and movement exercises are prescribed to be done throughout the day at set intervals to force the brain to complete the chemical changes.

Increasing reliance on vestibular information

Two things can happen when an inner ear starts acting up or loses function. A person may limit their activities to avoid symptoms and/or the brain may stop the bad information from arriving in the vestibular area of the brain (due to the so-called cerebellar clamp). Both these actions lead to increased reliance on vision and proprioception. During the acute period of illness this is a good thing but if it continues too long it becomes bad.

Vision is the most easily tricked of the three balance senses. If vision is used more than normal, problems misinterpreting the amount and direction of movement can occur. When vision gives information to the brain that doesn't agree with the vestibular and proprioceptive information there's a "sensory mismatch" resulting in symptoms that can be similar to seasickness. A confused brain is an unhappy brain and an unhappy brain can cause dizziness and nausea, even vomiting.

Some people get to the point of being unable to look at moving objects or confusing visual scenes without feeling sick. In this case exercises are prescribed to reduce the dependence on vision and improve the ability to look at movement. These exercises will include closing the eyes while standing still and walking with the eyes closed and may progress to looking at confusing or busy things as well as walking in a busy place like a mall (with the eyes open).

Overdependence on proprioception can also occur. In this case exercises begin by standing on something soft like a thick piece of foam (3" to 4" thick) and may progress to walking on highly padded carpeting or beach sand.

Becoming accustomed to bad vestibular information and/or symptoms

The idea behind this goal is that the brain will ignore bad information and the symptoms they bring when repeatedly exposed to it by a process called habituation. Exercises that bring on the symptoms are prescribed and done many times each day over weeks to months until the symptoms stop.

Increasing reliance on vision and proprioception (sensory substitution)

Usually when there's a loss of nearly all vestibular function in both ears the brain will automatically start to use vision and proprioception more for balance. This process can take a while to reach its peak with months and sometimes a year or two needed. Exercises can be prescribed to help this process go faster and be more complete.

Increasing muscle strength

The strength to carry out balance is just as important as the other parts of balance (joint flexibility, alertness, normal brain, normal spinal cord, experience and practice and vestibular information, vision and proprioception). Strengthening exercises can be prescribed if any areas of muscle weakness are found during the examination.

Increasing joint flexibility

Joint flexibility is just as important as muscle strength and all other parts of balance. The physical therapist can recommend flexibility exercises or other therapies if joint stiffness is found during the examination, particularly in the legs.

Improving the vestibulocular reflex

This reflex responsible for steady vision is disrupted by the loss of vestibular function or from bad vestibular information arriving in the brain. Exercises can be prescribed to help get as much use as possible from what remains of the VOR. They include things like staring at the small print on a business card taped to the wall while moving the head and can progress to watching a moving object while moving the head.

Balance practice and experience

Good balance requires practice and experience at many skills in many situations. After a vestibular loss or disruption the brain may need to gain experience and practice all over again at the skills and situations needed for daily life. Some people are successful at doing this on their own and others need help to get it done.

Alternative Form of Exercise

Tai chi, a Chinese exercise regimen, has been reported by one research group to improve balance in people with vestibular disorders. Most cities and large towns have Tai chi instructors and classes.

Sum Up

This treatment can help many people with a wide assortment of vestibular disorders by reducing symptoms and improving balance. Because vestibular disorders are a very specialized little area of health care a rehabilitation program should be set up and run by someone with thorough education and experience in the area who can figure out what a person needs, when they need it and how it can be provided.

Next

Surgery will be covered in the next chapter.

References and Reading List:

Alpini, D., Claussen, C.F., and Cesarani, A. *Vertigo and dizziness rehabilitation: the Mcs method.* New York: Springer Verlag, 1999.

Beidel, D.C., and Horak, F.B. "Behavior therapy for vestibular rehabilitation." *Journal of Anxiety Disorders,* 15:121-130, 2001.

Blakley, B.W. "Vestibular rehabilitation on a budget." *Journal of Otolaryngology,* 28(4):205-210, 1999.

Brandt, T.H., and Daroff, R.B. "Physical therapy for benign paroxysmal positional vertigo." *Archives of Otolaryngology-Head and Neck Surgery,* 106:484-485, 1980.

Cawthorne, T.E. "The physiological basis for head exercises." *Journal of the Chartered Society of Physiotherapy,* 29:106, 1944.

Cawthorne, T. "Vestibular injuries." *Proceedings of the Royal Society of Medicine,* 39:270-272, 1945.

Clendaniel, R.A., and Tucci, D.L. "Vestibular rehabilitation strategies in Meniere's disease." *Otolaryngologic Clinics of North America,* 30(6):1145-1158, 1997.

Cooksey, F.S. "Rehabilitation in vestibular injuries." *Proceedings of the Royal Society of Medicine,* 39:273-275, 1945.

Epley, J.M. "Canalith repositioning procedure." *Otolaryngology-Head and Neck Surgery*, 107(3):399-404, 1992.

Hahn, A., Sejna, I., Stolbova, K., and Cocek, A. "Visuo-vestibular biofeedback in patients with peripheral vestibular disorders." *Acta Otolaryngologica*, Supplement 545:88-91, 2001.

Hain, T.C., Fuller, L., Weil, L., and Kotsias, J. "Effects of T'ai Chi on Balance." *Archives of Otolaryngology-Head and Neck Surgery*, 125(11):1191-1195, 1999.

Herdman, S.J. *Vestibular rehabilitation*. Second edition. Philadelphia: F.A. Davis and Company, 2000.

Luxon, L.M., and Davies, R.A. *Handbook of vestibular rehabilitation*. San Diego: Singular Publishing Group, Inc., 1997.

McCabe, B.F. "Labyrinthine exercises in the treatment of diseases characterized by vertigo: their physiologic basis and methodology." *Laryngoscope*, 80:1429, 1970.

Norre, M.E., and DeWeerdt, W. "Treatment of vertigo based on habituation 2. Technique and results of habituation training." *Journal of Laryngology and Otology*, 94:971-977, 1980.

Shepard, N.T., and Telian, S.A. *Practical management of the balance disorder patient*. San Diego: Singular Publishing Group, 1996.

Telian, S.A., and Shepard, N.T. "Update on vestibular rehabilitation therapy." *Otolaryngologic Clinics of North America*, 29:357-71, 1996.

Chapter Fourteen
Surgery

The story on surgery for vestibular diseases isn't a simple one. Some vestibular disorders, like tumors, may require surgery while others, like vestibular neuronitis and ototoxicity, can't be helped at all with surgery. Most disorders fall in between with surgery mostly a treatment of last resort for the relief of certain types of severe vestibular symptoms.

Why not just go ahead and cut out a vestibular problem with surgery? Good question. Unfortunately the current state of vestibular knowledge isn't good enough to determine the exact area of microscopic damage, the inner ear is very small and encased in bone making surgery here difficult, surgically opening up the inner ear always places hearing and balance at huge risk for damage and the science doesn't exist to fix inner ear damage even if it could be located and reached easily.

Then why not just remove the entire inner ear? Taking out the inner ear creates a whole new set of problems like deafness not to mention problems with balance itself. It would also risk nerve damage leading to partial paralysis of the face and problems with taste.

Despite all of this, surgery can be the right treatment at times.

The Decision
Surgery isn't a quick fix or a sure thing; it's just one more treatment option (with a few more risks) to consider. If your problem is a tumor, perilymphatic fistula or cholesteatoma or the cause of your vestibular disorder can't be found and treated, if you have tried a number of medical treatments without any luck and if your vestibular symptoms are intolerable surgery might be the best choice.

A decision about surgery really boils down to thinking about the answers to two questions: Can the condition by treated with surgery? Should it be treated with surgery?

Can surgery help?
Whether or not a vestibular disorder is treatable with surgery can only be determined by an experienced ear doctor who has read a person's records then examined and tested them. They'll look at the symptoms, amount of disability, suffering, test results, diagnosis, hearing levels, if one ear or both ears are affected, what other treatments have been tried, how long the disorder has gone on, the age and if any other illnesses are also occurring.

Should surgery be done?

This question can only be answered by the person considering surgery, particularly if the surgery is solely for symptom relief (and not for a tumor and that sort of thing). They alone know how much they're suffering, how their life has been affected and how many medical treatments they've tried.

DO NOT have surgery if you don't trust your doctor, if you don't understand what you're getting into, if you don't understand the possible benefits of the surgery along with the risks or if your questions haven't been answered satisfactorily.

Some questions your doctor should answer for you include:

- Are you sure the problem is coming from the inner ear? How sure?
- Is the other ear OK?
- Are you sure surgery will help? How sure?
- Can something else be done instead of surgery?
- What are all the risks of the surgery and anesthesia?
- How many of these surgeries have you done?
- How many were successes?
- What do you consider success?
- How many people were made worse? In what way?
- What percent had complications and what were they? (Terms like rare or unlikely aren't good enough, try and get some numbers)
- What will you do for me if the surgery doesn't work or makes me worse?

Ask for the statistics for their patients, not statistics published by another surgeon. Make sure all your questions are answered, can be understood and seem logical. It might help to take someone along with you to the doctors' office for moral support and to help listen to the doctor. Look into your soul too. If you have surgery and a bad result occurs can you live with it? - or- Can you live with it if you don't make the effort to have surgery?

Making a decision like this is difficult. Take the time and energy to do it right. Clear your schedule and your mind and really think it through. Don't rush into surgery.

Risks of Surgery
All surgery has risk involved. How much risk depends on the person having the surgery, the type of anesthesia used, the type surgery, and the health care professionals doing it.

General Risks
Having other diseases
Some people are more at risk from surgery than others. Folks with serious disorders such as diabetes mellitus, heart disease, respiratory disease, history of having had a brain attack (stroke), undergoing treatment for blood clotting (particularly with a drug such as coumadin), liver disease, kidney disease or a system wide autoimmune disorder are at the highest risk. A specialist needs to know if a person has a serious illness or difficulties with healing, infection or bleeding, in addition to their vestibular disorder. Surgery should also be discussed with the PCP and other specialists being seen.

Anesthesia
Local anesthesia has the lowest risk of serious reactions. General anesthesia has more risk because multiple, potent drugs are used that circulate rapidly throughout the body. On occasion people have allergic or other bad reactions to these drugs, and very, very rarely can die from a reaction.

In addition to drugs, a breathing tube is inserted during general anesthesia that frequently causes a sore throat and on very rare occasion a fat lip or broken tooth.

Surgery

Every surgery has the risk of infection, excessive bleeding, or having the wrong thing cut or damaged. When something does go badly in ear surgery it usually affects hearing, balance, taste, or facial nerve function. Each surgery described later includes more information about its risk.

Health Care Professionals

Many times a person doesn't get much choice in the health care professionals they must deal with. Get yourself an experienced surgeon who only works with ears or inner ears, if you can. Sometimes talking to people who have had the surgery, particularly by the same surgeon, can be helpful in the selection. If your surgeon or their office staff can't help you, find a local support group or someone on the VEDA link list or perhaps people on the internet who have "been there, done that," to talk to.

Since you won't be able to choose a specific anesthesiologist ask your surgeon about the anesthesiologist or nurse anesthetist they use if you're concerned about this part of the surgery.

Balance Risks

This is such a complicated topic there are two versions here, the no frills and the in-depth.

No Frills

Some surgeries are designed to stop balance signals from leaving the ear and some have different goals. Either type surgery, at times, can lead to increased vestibular symptoms and/or decreased balance.

In-depth

Some surgeries attempt to fix a vestibular problem while others are designed to stop all balance signals from moving on to the brain. Either type of surgery can cause both balance symptoms and problems.

Even if ear surgery isn't intended to change balance signals the trauma of surgery might cause a temporary or permanent change anyway. The symptoms can be very low key, intolerable or anything in between.

There are two different types of permanent problems, lost function and frequently changing signals. Changing vestibular signals can make life pretty difficult with symptoms coming on far apart, very frequently or nearly constantly. Permanent loss of function can cause problems for a short while until the brain chemically compensates or can be long term if it doesn't.

After surgery designed to stop balance signals from arriving in the brain there will be a period of severe symptoms followed by a recuperation period and a return to normal (if the other ear is normal and the brain able to chemically compensate, that is).

The risk of this surgery is that the other ear really isn't normal and/or the brain can't chemically compensate for the change. If either is the case a person can be left with increased symptoms and a lot of difficulty moving around, particularly in the dark or on an angled surface.

A further risk is that the surgery will go well but the opposite ear will start having problems at a later time leaving a person with less balance function than if they had not undergone the surgery. If this happens there may also be more visual difficulties, possibly even bouncing vision (oscillopsia).

The Surgeries

Surgeries for vestibular symptoms aren't all done in the inner ear. They sometimes are also done on surrounding areas like the eardrum, middle ear, mastoid bone, internal auditory canal and the space around the brain.

Ear Drum

Most eardrum surgeries are performed for either eardrum or middle ear problems. Once in a while though, eardrum surgery will be done for a vestibular problem or symptoms.

Insertion of an ear tube (tympanostomy)

A tube with one end in the external ear canal and one end in the middle ear is inserted during this surgery. Adults usually have it done in the doctor's office using local anesthesia. Children usually require general anesthesia.

After local anesthesia is given a hole is made through the eardrum with a scalpel or LASER and a tube inserted. The tube is not stitched in place and most tubes will fall out months down the road. There are several models of tubes in use with some tubes staying in place longer then others.

Tubes come in a number of sizes and shapes. The T-shaped model can stay in place indefinitely while the others fall out over weeks to months.

This surgery isn't done very often for vestibular problems in the U.S. When it is, there are four reasons it might be done:

- To place medication into the middle ear from where it can travel to the inner ear
- As the first step in using the Meniett machine for treatment of Meniere's disease
- To get the air pressure on both sides of the ear drum to be the same (equalize)
- To limit movement of the ear drum

Some doctors will insert a Microwick through the tube and then give Decadron or gentamicin eardrops.

Because this surgery is usually done with local anesthesia it's low risk surgery. The most common problem that occurs is a failure of the hole to close back up on it's own once the tube is out. This occurs more frequently with the T-shaped models. If that happens it's usually treated successfully with a patch. Infections also occur on occasion.

After an ear tube insertion most people go immediately back to their usual activities only with restrictions on getting water into the ear canal while swimming and similar activities.

Tympanotomy

This surgical procedure moves the eardrum out of the way so a surgeon can put an instrument into the middle ear. It's done in the operating room under either local or general anesthesia.

An incision is made and the eardrum folded back on itself so it no longer covers the end of the ear canal. The surgeon can then put instruments into the middle ear to continue on with the rest of the surgery.

At the end of the surgery the eardrum is unfolded and put back into its proper place. The ear canal is then packed with both medication and a dressing that will stay in place for about a week.

Hearing is decreased for a while due to the dressing and because the surgery temporarily leaves fluids in the middle ear. It's important to keep water out of the ear canal after the surgery for as long as the surgeon instructs.

Whenever this surgery is done, no matter what the reason, there is a slight risk of eardrum damage or trauma to the little middle ear bones. This surgery, like all others, carries the risk of infection and complications from the anesthesia. When done by a qualified, experienced and skilled ear surgeon the risk is usually low.

This operation may be done as the first step in surgery to remove or repair the damage from a cholesteatoma, at the beginning of a perilymphatic fistula repair, or as the starting point for the seldom done transcanal labyrinthectomy. It can also be used to place drugs such as gentamicin into the middle ear.

The risks include infection, permanent hearing loss and changed taste (part of the nerve sending taste information from the tongue to the brain travels through the middle ear).

Middle Ear Surgeries

Like the eardrum surgeries, the vast majority of middle ear surgeries done by an ear surgeon aren't for vestibular problems or symptoms. There are, however, three surgeries that can improve vestibular problems in the right situation.

Even when done by a well-trained, experienced and skillful surgeon these middle ear surgeries still have a small risk of damage. Hearing may be lost and vestibular symptoms could possibly worsen from damage during the surgery itself or from a reaction to the surgery called serous labyrinthitis. Another risk is to the sense of taste. Part of the nerve responsible for the tongues ability to taste runs through the middle ear and can be injured. There's also the usual risk of infection.

These surgeries can cause swelling around the end of the eustachian tube so the ear may not pop or equalize the pressure on both sides of the eardrum for a while. A person should not fly, scuba dive or go into the mountains after this surgery without first asking their doctor. Water must not enter the ear canal for days to weeks after the surgery. Each surgeon will have his/her own set of post-operative instructions and most will include keeping water out of the ear canal for days to weeks after the surgery and some will restrict heavy lifting and pressure changes as well.

Endoscopy

A tympanotomy is done and a very small endoscope (A long, tube containing fiberoptics used to see inside the body) is inserted and the middle ear carefully examined.

Perilymphatic fistula repair

This surgery is done most often in folks who are rapidly loosing hearing, sometimes as an emergency surgery.

After a tympanotomy is done, fat or tissue patches are glued onto both the oval window and round window (membrane covered openings between the inner ear and middle ear) thought to be leaking. It's done in the operating room with either general or local anesthesia.

The tissue for the patch is taken from the external ear and the glue either comes pre-made from a manufacturer or is made from the person's own blood. Sometimes a bit of bone is removed from around the round window area of the middle ear at the beginning of this surgery.

Both the diagnosis and treatment of a perilymphatic fistula are a bit controversial. Some doctors do quite a few of these surgeries and others almost never do them.

Recuperation after a fistula repair may include a reduction in activities and avoiding pressure changes for several weeks while the ear heals completely.

Stapedectomy

A tympanotomy is done and the stapes bone is removed during this surgery. When done for otosclerosis a replacement stapes (stapes prosthesis) is also inserted.

This procedure is done most often for otosclerosis but can also be done if the stapes has been damaged from trauma or a cholesteatoma. In really rare situations it might also be done to help a perilymphatic fistula heal up.

Hearing is muffled for a while after the surgery due to the bandage and fluids in the ear made by the surgery.

This surgery isn't without risk. A severe hearing loss or deafness occurs 1% or more of the time. Serous labyrinthitis can occur and damage both the hearing and vestibular areas of the inner ear. If a perilymphatic fistula is created further surgery might be required. On rare occasion benign paroxysmal positional vertigo may be caused by this surgery. Luckily it can usually be helped with medical treatment.

Cholesteatoma removal

Middle ear surgery to remove a cholesteatoma or repair it's damage can also be done. The type and extent of the surgery is so different from one person to the next that a single description can't be given. Sometimes one surgery is done, other times multiple operations such as stapedectomy, perilymphatic fistula repair, and mastoidectomy are done. On rare occasion a labyrinthectomy might even be done to block vestibular symptoms.

Singular Neurectomy

This surgery is done to stop posterior semicircular canal information from flowing to the brain in someone with posterior canal benign paroxysmal positional vertigo (BPPV). The singular neurectomy is very, very rarely done because BPPV almost never requires surgery and when it does almost all surgeons use posterior semicircular canal plugging surgery instead.

Under local or general anesthesia, and after a tympanotomy is done, an instrument is inserted into the inner ear to destroy the singular nerve. A person may be awake during the surgery to tell the surgeon what type vestibular feelings they are having as the surgery goes along.

In addition to the other risks of doing a tympanotomy this surgery places hearing at more risk than insertion of an ear tube.

Inner Ear Surgeries

Unlike the eardrum and middle ear surgeries, inner ear surgeries are only done for vestibular problems.

Mastoidectomy

A mastoidectomy is done as the first step when performing endolymphatic sac surgery, labyrinthectomy, posterior semicircular canal plugging or vestibular nerve section. This surgery is also done to treat chronic middle ear infections and remove cholesteatomas. A mastoidectomy is a partial removal of the bone behind the ear called the mastoid bone. General anesthesia is used, some hair must be shaved from the area behind the ear, and a C-shaped incision is done that may require stitches and will leave a scar.

Depending on how the surgery is done a depression may be left behind the ear that interferes a bit with wearing glasses in some people. This area may also be sensitive to touch and pressure for months or more after the surgery. A procedure requiring more time and skill can be done to avoid a large depression—ask your surgeon about this if it's a concern.

After a mastoidectomy there's usually a large bandage over the ear that's wrapped around the forehead and back of the head.

No matter why a mastoidectomy is done there are some common problems after the surgery. Fluid may collect in the middle ear and cause reduced hearing for several days. Areas of numbness may occur on, and behind, the external ear that usually improves over time. The sense of taste can also be temporarily disrupted. The end of the eustachian tube may also be swollen shut causing sound distortion and possibly some pain, particularly while swallowing. Unexpected problems can occur as well including infection, hearing loss, disturbed vestibular function, increased tinnitus and facial nerve damage.

Endolymphatic Sac Surgeries
There are a number of surgeries in this category including endolymphatic sac decompression, endolymphatic sac shunt and endolymphatic sac valve insertion. All begin with a mastoidectomy and are followed by removal of bone until the endolymphatic sac is located.
Decompression
The endolymphatic sac is located and all the bone around it removed. It's believed this will improve circulation to the sac or allow it to expand so it can work better or hold more endolymphatic fluid.
Shunt
The endolymphatic sac is found, an opening made into it and either a premade straw-like tube or a piece of silastic sheeting inserted with the other end left in the mastoid space. In the past a small hole was made through the skull into the space around the brain where the end of the tube was placed.
Valve
In this version of the surgery a manufactured pressure release valve is implanted instead of the straw or sheeting. The idea here is that excess endolymphatic fluid will escape only as needed.

All of these procedures are done with general anesthesia as "same day surgery" which means showing up at the surgical center in the morning and leaving in the afternoon or early evening. The amount of pain experienced is usually minimal and most people can resume their usual activities a day or two after the surgery. Instructions after surgery usually include not shampooing the hair for a number of days.

In addition to the chance of failure this type surgery can also cause hearing loss (possibly even deafness), infection, serous labyrinthitis, persistent spinal fluid leak, an increase in vestibular symptoms, or facial nerve damage. According to published reports this surgery causes hearing loss or deafness in 5% of people having it done.

Some surgeons perform these surgeries regularly and others never do them because they feel that after a year or two people who have had the surgery are no better off than those who have not had it.

The success rates of published reports vary from 50 to 70%. A reduction in symptoms may not be immediate and might take several weeks.

Posterior semicircular canal plugging
This surgery is for benign paroxysmal positional vertigo (BPPV) of the posterior semicircular canal, the most common form of BPPV. It's not done very often because most cases of BPPV can be successfully treated without surgery.
A mastoidectomy is done and enough bone removed to see the posterior semicircular canal. A hole is drilled into the canal and bone chips inserted until the canal is totally plugged up.
The idea is that if the fluid in the canal can't move, symptoms won't happen. Most published accounts claim a nearly perfect success rate but there are people who have not been helped.
For the first few days or weeks after the surgery some people have problems with balance,

particularly during head movement. This clears up as they become more active or as they are treated with vestibular rehabilitation therapy. Most people can resume their usual activities quickly after the surgery.

Superior semicircular canal plugging

This surgery is done on rare occasion to treat superior semicircular canal dehiscence and is nearly identical to the posterior canal plugging procedure except it's the superior semicircular canal that's plugged.

Labyrinthectomy

This surgery is done to stop attacks of violent vertigo in folks who have lost all, or nearly all, hearing in one ear. It isn't quite as straightforward as the name implies. The word labyrinthectomy literally means "removal of the labyrinth" but the entire labyrinth isn't removed.

There are two general ways it can be done; with an incision behind the ear (i.e. after first doing a mastoidectomy) or through the middle ear (after first doing a tympanotomy). The first surgery is called the transmastoid approach and the second the transcanal approach.

In the transmastoid approach all five balance parts of the inner ear; the contents inside the ampulla of the posterior, horizontal, and anterior semicircular canals and the maccula of the utricle and saccule, are removed. This is done by drilling through the temporal bone to each of the five spots and scraping or sucking out the cells in these microscopic areas.

There is another version of the transmastoid surgery called the translabyrinthine vestibular nerve section. After removing all five balance areas further surgery is done to cut the vestibular nerve within the internal auditory canal.

The second general method of doing a labyrinthectomy is a transcanal labyrinthectomy. In this surgery a tympanotomy is done, the oval window pierced and a vacuum like device used to suck out the contents of the inner ear. This is done blindly with no guarantee that all five balance hair cell areas of the inner ear will be completely sucked out.

In all versions of the labyrinthectomy hearing is lost due to the trauma of the surgery.

Following the surgery, symptoms range from nothing more than a bit of pain when lifting the head up to horrific vertigo and vomiting for days that must be treated with drugs. People missing the most vestibular function before surgery have the least amount of vestibular symptoms after the surgery and those with the most vestibular function left, at the time of the surgery, have the most symptoms.

Some doctors begin vestibular rehabilitation therapy the day after surgery to help the brain chemically compensate. Recuperation to the point of returning to work and "normal" activities varies, a lot. It can take a week for some people and several months for others. For a few people this may never be complete.

The risks of this surgery include facial nerve damage that could cause permanent drooping of the face and eyelid on one side of the face, an increase in tinnitus, persistent spinal fluid leak, infection, hematoma or collection of blood, taste disturbance, and dry mouth.

Another possible bad outcome is that the vertigo might not be eliminated and/or the brain may not be able to compensate for the total loss of balance function on the one side.

Head Surgery
Vestibular nerve section

In this surgery the vestibular branch of the vestibulocochlear nerve is cut to stop the flow of balance information from the ear to the brain. The problem causing the violent attacks of spontaneous vertigo is not fixed, instead the message is prevented from reaching the brain.

It's usually done in people who still have some hearing in the problem ear. If nearly all hearing is gone a labyrinthectomy is more commonly done.

This is one of the more serious vestibular surgeries because the nerve is cut very near the brain. Despite this, the surgery is relatively safe with death unheard of these days. The hearing and facial nerves are more at risk than the brain in this surgery. The most likely complication from the surgery is further loss of hearing. Other possibilities include facial nerve damage and spinal fluid leak.

There are several versions of this surgery including: the retrolabyrinthine, middle fossa, retrosigmoid, suboccipital and the combination retrolabyrinthine/retrosigmoid. Most of these begin with a mastoidectomy followed by further drilling until the vestibulocochlear nerve is found in the space near the brain. Many times the empty space left by this surgery is filled with fat and other tissue from a person's own abdomen or the area behind the ear.

Following the surgery, symptoms range from nothing more than feeling a bit feverish and having some pain when lifting the head up to horrific vertigo and vomiting lasting for days. People missing the most vestibular function before surgery have the least amount of vestibular symptoms after the surgery and those with the most vestibular function left at the time of the surgery have the most symptoms.

Cutting the nerve carrying balance information sounds pretty straight forward, right? Well, the hearing and balance nerve travel part of the way to the brain within the same covering and figuring out where one ends and the other begins is not always possible. This surgery does not always eliminate the vertigo, possibly because the nerve hasn't been fully cut.

Technical point: A paper describing the vestibulocochlear nerve was published in 1940: Rasmussen, A.T. "Studies of the VIIIth cranial nerve of man." *Laryngoscope*, 50:57-83.

Since transtympanic gentamicin came onto the scene the number of vestibular nerve sections being done has dropped.

Microvascular Decompression
In this surgery an opening is made into the space around the brain and a pad placed between the vestibulocochlear nerve and the blood vessel pressing on it.

This is another of the more serious vestibular surgeries because it takes place very near the brain. Despite this, the surgery is relatively safe when done by a skilled surgeon who has a great deal of surgical experience.

Where the incision is made will depend upon the location of the vessel and the personal preference of the surgeon. How someone feels and how well he or she recovers after the surgery varies quite a bit.

Acoustic Neuroma removal
An acoustic neuroma is a tumor that grows from the vestibular branch of the vestibulocochlear nerve. Not only does surgical removal involve cutting out part of the vestibular nerve it may also be necessary to cut the hearing nerve and the facial nerve during the surgery.

Even if the hearing and facial nerves are not cut they can be damaged severely. The chance of losing hearing and/or facial function depends upon the position and size of the tumor, how well equipped the hospital's operating room is and the skill and experience of the surgeon.

Some surgeons are better at saving function than others so time should be spent looking for the best surgeon. Join the Acoustic Neuroma Association and find people who have had the surgery and talk to them about their experience and doctors. Ask what they would do differently if given the chance. Acoustic Neuroma Association, www.anausa.org and 600 Peachtree Suite 108, Cumming, GA 30014 770-205-8211

Loss of all hearing in one ear means a person can't figure out what direction sound is coming from. If someone yells come this way, what way this way is, will not be immediately known. It also means only one ear can be used during a long phone conversation and when being seated at a table one must figure out where to sit so they can hear everything.

Reduced facial function means an eyelid on the side with the loss won't blink or close all the way. A smile will only happen halfway with just one side of the mouth moving.

These changes can be lived with if they are the only option but if they can be saved it's worth the effort even if it means traveling a great distance and possibly spending more money.

After this surgery symptoms range from nothing more than a bit of pain when lifting the head up to horrific vertigo and vomiting for days. People missing the most vestibular function before their surgery have the least amount of vestibular symptoms after the surgery and those with a lot of vestibular function left at the time of the surgery have the most symptoms.

Some people are able to just resume their prior activities very quickly after surgery while others will require vestibular rehabilitation therapy to get going. Prolonged problems with headaches after the surgery can also occur.

For in-depth, specific information about all the details of these surgeries, what's cut and that sort of thing there are many articles, a few books and a web page with pictures and diagrams for those with a strong stomach at www.earsurgery.org/

Sum Up
Surgery is available for some vestibular problems but usually isn't the first treatment offered.

Next
Individual diseases are described beginning with the next chapter.

References and Reading List:
Agrawal, S.K., and Parnes, L.S. "Human experience with canal plugging." *Annals of New York Academy of Science*, 942:300-305, 2001.

Arenberg, I. K., and Graham, M. *Treatment options for Meniere's Disease: endolymphatic sac surgery: do it or don't do it and why.* San Diego, CA, Singular Publishing Group, 1998.

Brackmann, D. E., Shelton, C., and Arriaga, M. A. *Otologic surgery.* Second edition. Philadelphia: W. B. Saunders Company. 2001.

Kerr, A. G. "Emotional investments in surgical decision making." *Journal of Laryngology and Otology*, 116:575-579, 2002.

Magnan, J., and Sanna, M. *Endoscopy in neuro-otology.* New York: Thieme Medical Publishing, 1999.

Nadol, J. B., and Schuknecht, H.F. *Surgery of the ear and temporal bone.* New York: Raven Press, 1992.

Reid, C.B., Eisenberg, R., Halmagyi, G.M., and Fagan, P.A. "The outcome of vestibular nerve section for intractable vertigo: the patient's point of view." *Laryngoscope*, 106:1553-1556, 1996.

Silverstein, H. "Use of a new device, the MicroWick, to deliver medication to the inner ear." *Ear Nose Throat Journal,* 78(8):595-598, 600, 1999.

Yung, M.W. "The use of middle ear endoscopy: has residual cholesteatoma been eliminated?" *Journal of Laryngology and Otology,* 115(12):958-961, 2001.

Chapter Fifteen
Acoustic Neuroma

This is a benign tumor of the vestibular branch of the vestibulocochlear nerve. Tumors aren't a very common cause of vestibular symptoms but when present in an adult with inner ear dizziness symptoms it's usually a benign acoustic neuroma. According to the Acoustic Neuroma Association acoustic neuromas large enough to cause inner ear symptoms occur in about one person in 100,000.

A more technically correct name for this tumor is vestibular schwannoma since the tumor almost always begins in the schwann cells of the vestibular branch of the vestibulocochlear nerve. Other names in use are acoustic neurinoma and acoustic neurilemoma.

There are two forms of acoustic neuroma, inherited (bilateral hereditary) and non-inherited (unilateral sporadic). The inherited form is also referred to as Neurofibromatosus type II (NF-2). It is the nastier of the two because it goes on to involve both ears. Luckily it is also the more rare occurring in only 5% of all people with acoustic neuroma.

Because these tumors grow within the tiny tunnel carrying the hearing, balance and facial nerve the symptoms revolve around these functions. Hearing loss on one side, ringing in the ear, vague feelings of unsteadiness or imbalance are the most common symptoms and might be accompanied by facial weakness.

The non-hereditary acoustic neuroma generally grows slowly with dramatic symptoms such as vertigo and vomiting occurring in only about 10-20% of the cases. Unsteadiness, particularly in the dark, is the more common vestibular symptom occurring in about half the people with the tumor.

This tumor may not be cancerous but it is still a very serious condition that can cause life-altering and life-threatening damage if allowed to grow too big. When large, it can press on the brain causing neurological symptoms such as trouble swallowing and speaking.

These tumors begin growing in the internal auditory canal (the tunnel between the inner ear and brain through which the hearing, balance and one facial movement nerve pass) and may grow to the point of pressing against the brain itself. These tumors generally grow slowly. Loss of vestibular function brings on dramatic symptoms such as vertigo and vomiting in only about 10-20% of the cases.

The ABR hearing test was at one time THE method for diagnosing acoustic neuromas but since MRI's with gadolineum enhancement came on the scene in the 1980's they have taken over that position. There continue to be technical reasons for using the ABR in the diagnostic process so your doctor might ask you to undergo both.

Removal is the most common treatment offered to younger people and those in the best health. There are two methods, one surgical and the other radiological. Stereotactic radiation is the less disruptive of the two but not every tumor can be dealt with in this way (the size of the tumor and its location must be considered).

In older folks or those in ill health waiting and watching may be the treatment approach taken in dealing with an acoustic neuroma. The watching is done in part by measuring tumor growth with an MRI every few months.

Surgical Removal
In addition to the usual risks of any surgery, removal of an acoustic neuroma can also cause hearing loss, facial paralysis, chronic headaches and balance disturbances. The best hearing results occur when the tumor is small and the surgeon is trained, experienced and highly skilled in their removal and the operating room has all the latest equipment. Ask your surgeon about his/her track record in this area.

Loss of vestibular function on one side isn't usually as large an issue as hearing and facial function because over the days to weeks after surgery the brain learns to use information from the opposite ear to perform balance. Some people do have trouble with this change and may be helped through it with vestibular rehabilitation therapy.

For more information and/or to meet up with other people who have acoustic neuromas check out the Acoustic Neuroma Association at www.anausa.org or 600 Peachtree, Suite 108, Cumming, GA 30014 770-205-8211. Joining the ANA is also a way to locate doctors experienced in treating these tumors and increasing the chance for the best outcome.

References and Reading List:
Belal, A. "Is cochlear implantation possible after acoustic tumor removal?" *Otology and Neurotology,* 22:497-500, 2001.

Briggs, R.J., Fabinyi, G., and Kaye, A.H. "Current management of acoustic neuromas: review of surgical approaches and outcomes." *Journal of Clinical Neuroscience,* 7(6):521-526, 2000.

Brophy, B.P. "Acoustic neuroma—surgery or radiosurgery?" *Stereotactic Functional Neurosurgery,* 74(3-4):121-128, 2000.

Hoistad, D.L., Melnik, G., Mamikoglu, B., Battista, R., O'Connor, C.A., and Wiet, R.J. "Update on conservative management of acoustic neuroma." *Otology and Neurotology,* 22:682-685, 2001.

Kaylie, D.M., Gilbert, E., Horgan, M.A., Delashaw, J.B., and McMenomey, S.O. "Acoustic neuroma surgery outcomes." *Otology and Neurotology,* 22(5):686-689, 2001.

Levo, H., Blomstedt, G., and Pyykko, I. "Is hearing preservation useful in vestibular schwannoma surgery?" *Annals of Otology, Rhinology and Laryngology,* 111(5 Pt 1):392-396, 2002.

Levo, H., Blomstedt, G., Hirvonen, T., and Pyykko, I. "Causes of persistent postoperative headache after surgeryfor vestibular schwannoma." *Clinical Otolaryngology,* 26:401-406, 2001.

Magliulo, G., Zardo, F., Damico, R., Varacalli, S., and Forino, M. "Acoustic neuroma: postoperative quality of life." *Journal of Otolaryngology,* 29(6):344-347, 2000.

Mamikoglu, B., Wiet, R.J., and Esquivel, C.R. "Translabyrinthine approach for the management of large and giant vestibular schwannomas." *Otology and Neurotology, 23*(2):224-227, 2002.

Perry, B.P., Gantz, B.J., and Rubinstein, J.T. "Acoustic neuromas in the elderly." *Otology and Neurotology,* 22(3):389-391, 2001.

Petit, J.H., Hudes, R.S., Chen, T.T., Eisenberg, H.M., Simard, J.M., and Chin, L.S. "Reduced-dose radiosurgery for vestibular schwannomas." *Neurosurgery, 49*(6):1299-1306; discussion 1306-1307, 2001.

Pothula, V.B., Lesser, T., Mallucci, C., May, P., and Foy, P. "Vestibular schwannomas in children." *Otology and Neurotology, 22*(6):903-907, 2001.

Ruckenstein, M.J., Harris, J.P., Cueva, R.A., Prioleau, G., and Alksne, J. "Pain subsequent to resection of acoustic neuromas via suboccipital and translabyrinthine approaches." *American Journal of Otology,* 17:620-624, 1996.

Sluyter, S., Graamans, K., Tulleken, C.A., and Van Veelen, C.W. "Analysis of the results obtained in 120 patients with large acoustic neuromas surgically treated via the translabyrinthine-transtentorial approach." *Journal of Neurosurgery,* 94(1):61-66, 2000.

Swan, I.R. "Is early management of acoustic neuroma important? "*Journal of the Royal Society of Medicine,* 93(12):614-617, 2000.

Warrick, P., Bance, M., and Rutka, J. "The risk of hearing loss in non-growing, conservatively managed acoustic neuromas." *American Journal of Otology,* 20:758-762, 1999.

Wiet, R.J., Mamikoglu, B., Odom, L., and Hoistad, D.L. "Long-term results of the first 500 cases of acoustic neuroma surgery." *Otolaryngology-Head and Neck Surgery,* 124:645-651, 2001.

Chapter Sixteen
Arnold-Chiari Malformation Type I

In this problem a part of the brain grows abnormally long and forces it's way into the foramen magnum, an opening at the bottom of the skull, that normally contains only the spinal cord. In addition, some people with Arnold-Chiari have other malformations usually involving the neck bones.

Technical point: The cerebellar tonsils protrude abnormally down into the foramen magnum in Arnold-Chiari malformation type I.

A Chiari malformation can create vestibular and other inner ear symptoms in three different ways: Direct pressure on the vestibular areas of the brain, increased fluid pressure throughout the brain and increased pressure sent into the inner ear through the cochlear aqueduct. (A tunnel traveling from the subarachnoid space around the brain into a perilymph fluid containing area of the inner ear).

The inner ear symptoms it can cause include hearing loss, tinnitus, ear pressure/pain, disequilibrium, imbalance and vertigo. These can be fairly constant or may come and go.

What typically sets this disorder apart from pure vestibular disorders is the presence of symptoms commonly seen from a brain under abnormal pressure. These pressure symptoms can include numb body areas, pain, headache, muscle weakness, and visual difficulties such as loss of areas of vision, visual floaters, sleep apnea, trouble swallowing, fainting, urinary difficulties, decreased gag reflex, tremors, and pain behind the eyes.

It's common for people with this disorder to experience inner ear symptoms but it's VERY unusual for Arnold-Chiari Malformation Type I to cause inner ear symptoms and nothing else. Arnold-Chiari malformation type I symptoms usually begin in young adulthood and may go on for 5 to 10 years before the correct diagnosis is made. The symptoms appear for the first time after trauma in about 20% of people diagnosed with it.

The diagnosis is usually finalized with an MRI of the brain. There is a bit of controversy about how much abnormal lengthening of the brain is needed to create symptoms and make the diagnosis. This argument literally comes down to millimeters measured on an MRI with a ruler. If the lengthening is less than 5 mm most doctors feel it can't produce symptoms, if 5mm or more they feel symptoms are possible.

Treatment is aimed at reducing the pressure on the brain and it's surrounding structures. In some people this can be done with drugs such as the diuretic Diamox (acetozolamide). In others a tube may be surgically implanted to release pressure and sometimes, serious surgery on the skull itself may be needed to reduce the pressure on the brain.

If you have this disorder or think you might, there are several organizations you can get information and moral support from:

In the U.S.:
American Syringomyelia Alliance Project, Inc.
www.asap4sm.com
P. O. Box 1586
Longview, Texas 75606-1586
Phone: 903-236-7079
Fax: 903-757-7456
1-800-ASAP-282

World Arnold-Chiari Malformation Association (WACMA)
www.pressenter.com/~wacma/
31 Newtown Woods Road,
Newtown Square
Philadelphia, PA 19073

In Canada:
Canadian Syringomyelia Network
69 Penny Crescent Markham,
Ontario L3P5X7
(905) 471-8278

In the UK:
United Kingdom Arnold-Chiari and Syringomyelia association
www.soft.net.uk/stregawarlock/syringom.htm#OI

References and Reading List:

Ahmmed, A.U., Mackenzie, I., Das, V.K., Chatterjeem, S., and Lye, R.H. "Audio-vestibular manifestations of Chiari malformation and outcome of surgical decompression: a case report." *Journal of Laryngology and Otology, 110*(11):1060-1064, 1996.

Albers, F.W., and Ingels, K.J. "Otoneurological manifestations in Chiari—I malformation." *Journal of Laryngology and Otology, 107*(5):441-443, 1993.

Chait, G. E., and Barber, H. O. "Arnold-Chiari malformation—some otoneurological features." *Journal of Otolaryngology, 8*(1):65-70, 1979.

Galvex, M.J., Rodrigo, J.J., Liesa, R.F., Gonzalez, E.A., Garrido, C.M., Samperiz, L.C., and Tajada, J.P. "Otorhinolaryngologic manifestations in Chiari malformation." *American Journal of Otolaryngology,* 23(2):99-104, 2002.

Hendrix, R.A., Bacon, C.K., and Sclafani, A.P. "Chiari-I malformation associated with asymmetric sensorineural hearing loss." *Journal of Otolaryngology, 21*(2):102-107, 1992.

Kumar, A. Patni, A.H., and Charbel, F. "The Chiari I Malformation and the neurotologist." *Otology and Neurotology*, 23:727-735, 2002.

Johnson, G.D., Harbaugh, R.E., and Lenz, S.B. "Surgical decompression of Chiari I malformation for isolated progressive sensorineural hearing loss." *American Journal of Otology*, 15(5):634-638, 1994.

Milhorat, T.H., Chou, M.W., Trinidad, E.M., Kula, R.W., Mandell, M., Wolpert, C., and Speer, M.C. "Chiari I malformation redefined: clinical and radiographic findings for 364 symptomatic patients." *Neurosurgery*, 44(5):1005-1017, 1999.

Samii, C., Mobius, E., Weber, W., Heienbrok, H.W., and Berlit, P. "Pseudo Chiari type I malformation secondary to cerebrospinal fluid leakage." *Journal of Neurology*, 246(3):162-164, 1999.

Sinclair, N., Assaad, N., and Johnston, I. "Pseudotumour cerebri occurring in association with the Chiari malformation." *Journal of Clinical Neuroscience*, 9(1):99-101, 2002.

Sperling, N.M., Franco, R.A. Jr., and Milhorat, T.H. "Otologic manifestations of Chiari I malformation." *Otology and Neurotology*, 22(5):678-681, 2001.

Stovner, L.J. "Headache associated with the Chiari type I malformation." *Headache*, 33(4):175-181, 1993.

Weber, P.C., and Cass, S.P. "Neurotologic manifestations of Chiari I malformation." *Otolaryngology-Head and Neck Surgery*, 109(5):853-860, 1993.

Yoshimi, A., Nomura, K., and Furune, S. "Sleep apnea syndrome associated with a type I Chiari malformation." *Brain Development*, 24(1):49-51, 2002.

Chapter Seventeen
Benign Paroxysmal Positional Vertigo (BPPV)

Quite a mouthful isn't it? Here's a break down of the name:

Benign: Isn't caused by a serious illness such as a brain tumor
Paroxysmal: Comes on very suddenly
Positional: Happens in certain head positions
Vertigo: A feeling of movement that isn't actually occurring or is occurring differently then what is felt

This disorder is also sometimes referred to as benign positional vertigo, or benign paroxysmal positional nystagmus.

So, this is vertigo originating from the inner ear that occurs suddenly in certain head positions. It's probably the disorder most commonly seen by inner ear balance experts in their offices.

The theory behind the symptoms in this disorder is that debris break loose from the utricle and float around in one or another of the semicircular canals or gets stuck on a structure within a semicircular canal called the cupula. This debris is thought to be the calcium carbonate otoliths that some doctors refer to as ear rocks.

BPPV is more common in older folks but can occur in anyone. The cause is never found in half the people who develop it and is more likely to remain unknown in older people. Trauma is the most common cause in younger people. It can also occur in people with other vestibular disorders like vestibular neuronitis, ototoxicity and Meniere's disease. Theories of other causes include viral infection, autoimmune reaction and genetic factors.

This disorder comes in several types. It can affect any of the three semicircular canals, (anterior, horizontal or posterior) singly or in combination. The vertigo may be present for seconds at a time once in a while or symptoms of one sort or another may be present much of the time. It can occur for days, weeks, months or even years and the severity can vary a lot.

BPPV can be classified by both the timing and the severity of symptoms.

Timing

Self-limiting BPPV: Stops on its own in weeks or months
Relapsing/remitting: Comes and goes over weeks to years
Persistent BPPV: Doesn't go away without surgical intervention

Severity

Mild BPPV: Occasional vertigo with head positioning and no symptoms in-between episodes.

Moderate BPPV: Vertigo occurs every time a particular head position is assumed and there may be symptoms in-between episodes such as lightheadedness

Extreme BPPV: Almost all head movement produces vertigo with symptoms such as nausea and lightheadedness present all the time.

By far the most common form of BPPV is self-limiting posterior semicircular canal BPPV with mild to moderate symptoms caused by the floating debris.

In this form of BPPV a person usually has strong, revolving vertigo when rolling onto one side in bed and/or when putting the head back to look up, like towards the top shelf in the kitchen. The vertigo lasts less than one minute and then stops, even if a person stays in the bad position. No vestibular symptoms occur between episodes.

Surprisingly there is a slam-dunk test for posterior canal BPPV, the Dix-Hallpike maneuver. In this test a person is moved rapidly from a sitting position to lying down with the head lower than the body and turned a bit to the side and while the eyes are watched. A doctor can even perform it right in their office without any sophisticated equipment but many prefer to have a technician do it as part of the ENG battery of tests.

The news gets even better about this disorder. In addition to a slam-dunk diagnostic test there are also a few relatively easy treatments available that don't require either drugs or surgery and may only require one or two further office visits to complete.

Two treatments, the canalith repositioning procedure (also called the Epley maneuver) and the Semont maneuver are both available. Without getting into specifics I'll just say both treatments involve moving the head and body in ways that help the loose debris float out of the semicircular canal. In addition some doctors also use a vibrator during the canalith repositioning maneuver. Unfortunately these treatments are the least effective in people with more than one vestibular disorder. When done by a well educated, trained and skilled professional these treatments do the trick 80% or more of the time.

The anterior semicircular canal is affected in about 4% of BPPV cases with symptoms similar to the posterior canal variety. This one can also be diagnosed using the Dix-Hallpike maneuver but the interpretation is slightly more complicated than posterior BPPV and requires more experience. This problem can also be treated with a canalith repositioning procedure.

Horizontal semicircular canal BPPV is the least common type. Vertigo of short duration occurs when rolling onto either side in bed and when shaking the head in the "no" direction. Some people also have additional symptoms in-between episodes including the feeling of walking on pillows, unsteadiness and nausea.

Testing for horizontal canal BPPV is not standard so the disorder may go undiagnosed. The test involves watching the eyes or recording their movement while putting the head and body through a number of movements.

If movement treatments don't work and the symptoms are disabling, surgery may be offered. The surgery in widest use is the canal plugging procedure in which the posterior semicircular canal is plugged with bone and tissue to stop the otoliths from floating around. Another older, more technically difficult surgery, is the singular neurectomy in which the branch of the vestibular nerve sending signals from the posterior semicircular canal to the brain is cut.

References and Reading List:

Atacan, E., Sennaroglu, L., Genc, A., and Kaya, S. "Benign paroxysmal positional vertigo after stapedectomy." *Laryngoscope*, 111(7):1257-1259, 2001.

Brantberg, K., and Bergenius, J. "Treatment of anterior benign paroxysmal positional vertigo by canal plugging: a case report." *Acta Otolaryngologica*, 122(1):28-30, 2002.

Epley, J.M. "The canalith repositioning procedure: for treatment of benign paroxysmal positional vertigo." *Otolaryngology-Head and Neck Surgery*, 107(3):399-404, 1992.

Epley, J.M. "Human experience with canalith repositioning maneuvers." *Annals of the New York Academy of Science*, 942:179-191, 2001.

Gacek, R.R., and Gacek, M.R. "The three faces of vestibular ganglionitis." *Annals of Otology, Rhinology and Laryngology*, 111(2):103-114, 2002.

Girardi, M., and Konrad, H.R. "Management of benign paroxysmal positional vertigo." *Official Journal of the Society of Otorhinolaryngology-Head and Neck Nursing*, 14(2):25-30, 1996.

Gizzi, M., Ayyagari, S., and Khattar, V. "The familial incidence of benign paroxysmal positional vertigo." *Acta Otolaryngologica*, 118(6):774-777, 1998.

Harada, K., Oda, M., Yamamoto, M., Nomura, T., Ohbayashi, S., and Kitsuda, C. "A clinical observation of benign paroxysmal positional vertigo after vestibular neuronitis (VN)." *Acta Otolaryngologica*, Supplement 503:61-63, 1993.

Haynes, D.S., Resser, J.R., Labadie, R.F., Girasole, C.R., Kovach, B.T., Scheker, L.E., and Walker, D.C. "Treatment of benign positional vertigo using the Semont maneuver: efficacy in patients presenting without nystagmus." *Laryngoscope*, 112(5):796-801, 2002.

Hughes, C.A., and Proctor, L. "Benign paroxysmal positional vertigo." *Laryngoscope*, 107(5):607-613, 1997.

Lanska, D.J., and Remler, B. "Benign paroxysmal positioning vertigo: classic descriptions, origins of the provocative positioning technique, and conceptual developments." *Neurology*, 48(5):1167-1177, 1997.

Li, J.C., Epley, J.M., and Weinberg, L. "Cost-effective management of benign positional vertigo using canalith repositioning." *Otolaryngology-Head and Neck Surgery*, 122(3):334-339, 2000.

Modugno, G.C., Pirodda, A., Ferri, G.G., Montana, T., Rasciti, L., and Ceroni, A.R. "A relationship between autoimmune thyroiditis and benign paroxysmal positional vertigo?" *Medical Hypotheses*, 54(4):614-615, 2000.

Monobe, H., Sugasawa, K., and Murofushi, T. "The outcome of the canalith repositioning procedure for benign paroxysmal positional vertigo: are there any characteristic features of treatment failure cases?" *Acta Otolaryngologica*, Supplement 545:38-40, 2001.

Nagarkar, A.N., Gupta, A.K., and Mann, S.B "Psychological findings in benign paroxysmal positional vertigo and psychogenic vertigo." *Journal of Otolaryngology*, 29(3):154-158, 2000.

Sherman, D., and Massoud, E.A. "Treatment outcomes of benign paroxysmal positional vertigo." *Journal of Otolaryngology*, 30(5):295-299, 2001.

Tusa, R.J. "Benign paroxysmal positional vertigo." *Current Neurology Neuroscience Report*, 1(5):478-485, 2001.

Chapter Eighteen
Benign Paroxysmal Vertigo of Childhood

Vestibular problems don't occur in children very often but when they do strike this is the most common. It usually hits between the ages of 1 and 4, but there are reports of kids as old as 12 having it.

Important note: This is benign paroxysmal vertigo of childhood, not benign paroxysmal positional vertigo.

Vertigo and/or disequilibrium begins suddenly is these kids. In addition to the vertigo they can also have nausea, vomiting, nystagmus, flushing and visual disturbances. It's so sudden and scary many kids yell out in fear when an episode starts. They may not be able to walk or even stand up and may crouch or cling to a parent during an episode. Episodes usually last from minutes to hours but attacks for 24 hours or greater have been reported in one or two children.

Note: Hearing loss, ringing in the ears and loss of consciousness are NOT part of this disorder.

Migraine is the leading theory for the cause of this disorder. It even has an International Headache Society classification number, 1.5.1

This diagnosis is usually made if the history and symptoms are a match and if no other cause for the symptoms can be found. Vestibular tests may be done to help rule out some conditions but there are no specific test results for benign paroxysmal vertigo of childhood. Because children don't usually have vestibular disorders non-vestibular tests such as an EEG, MRI and CT scans may be done to look for non-vestibular explanations. Most vestibular and hearing tests can be done on children but it requires them to cooperate during the testing, something a small child may not be able to do.

If your doctor is having trouble making a diagnosis because they haven't seen an attack, videotape your child during one. Be sure to film their eyes too.

There are no treatment studies so each doctor is kind of on their own in this area. Some doctors may suggest a wait and see or they'll outgrow it approach. Others might suggest a diet change to remove anything with tyramine from their diet. Anti-serotonin and anti-prostaglandin drugs may also be prescribed. If episodes last hours at a time vestibular suppressant drugs may be used. If vomiting lasts a long time anti-nausea drugs and IV fluids might be needed. Ask your doctor if a home fluid replacement like Pedialyte would help replace fluids after vomiting.

Keep the child safe during an episode by not allowing them to bang into things or fall. Don't allow a toddler with this disorder to roam around the neighborhood unsupervised. If the child goes to daycare or school discuss the situation fully with supervisory personnel.

The prognosis is one of those good news/bad news types. The good news is these episodes usually go on for a year or two and stop as mysteriously as they appeared leaving no permanent physical damage. The bad news is some of these kids go on to develop "regular" migraines, an outcome more common when a family member also has a history of migraines.

References and Reading List:

Al-Twaijri, W.A., and Shevell, M.I. "Pediatric migraine equivalents: occurrence and clinical features in practice." *Pediatric Neurology, 26(5):365-368, 2002.*

Baloh, R.W., and Honrubia, V. "Childhood onset of benign positional vertigo." *Neurology,* 50(5):1494-1496, 1998.

Barabas, G., Matthews, W.S., and Ferrari, M. "Childhood migraine and motion sickness." *Pediatrics,* 72:188-190, 1983.

Basser, L.S. "Benign paroxysmal vertigo of childhood: a variety of vestibular neuronitis." *Brain, 87*:141-152, 1964.

Cass, S.P., Furman, J.M., Ankerstjerne, K., Balaban, C., Yetiser, S., and Aydogan B. "Migraine-related vestibulopathy." *Annals of Otology, Rhinology, and Laryngology,* 106(3):182-189, 1997.

Drigo, P., Carli, G., and Laverda, A.M. "Benign paroxysmal vertigo of childhood." *Brain Development,* (1):38-41, 2001.

Eviatar, L. "Dizziness in children." *Otolaryngologic Clinics of North America,* 27(3):557-570, 1994.

Herraiz, C., Calvin, F.J., Tapia, M.C., de Lucas, P., and Arroyo, R. "The migraine: benign paroxysmal vertigo of childhood complex." *International Tinnitus Journal,* 5(1):50-52, 1999.

Lanzi, G., Balottin, U., Fazzi, E., Tagliasacchi, M., Manfrin, M., and Mira, E. "Benign paroxysmal vertigo of childhood: a long-term follow-up." *Cephalalgia,* 14(6):458-460, 1994.

Tusa, R.J., Saada, A.A., and Niparko, J.K. "Dizziness in Childhood." *Journal of Child Neurology,* 9(3):261-274, 1994.

Chapter Nineteen
Cervical Vertigo

Cervical or neck vertigo is more formally called cervicogenic vertigo. This is a shadowy disorder because there's no physical evidence to prove it exists—no X-Ray, no vestibular test changes, nothing that can be found with surgery, a physical change can't even be found after death (when all the parts of the neck and inner ear can be examined, completely, without fear of causing damage). Many times reasonable, alternative explanations for the symptoms exist as well.

So what is it? It's a theory that vestibular symptoms can be caused by a problem with the neck. Although cervical vertigo can't be seen or tested for, there's strong anatomical proof that the neck is involved in balance. The neck receives muscle adjustment signals from the inner ear balance areas via the brain and sends head position information up to the brain to help it make decisions about movement and our position in space. This occurs via the vestibulocollic reflex (VCR) and the cervicocollic reflex (CCR).

Another neck reflex, the cervicocular reflex (COR), exists and may play a very small role in maintaining clear vision. (As you might remember the VOR is the major player in keeping vision clear during head movement).

It stands to reason that change in these neck reflexes would lead to symptoms and/or functional difficulties.

Symptoms said to come from cervical vertigo are a swimming sensation in the head, disequilibrium, stiff neck, pain in the neck, pain in the upper back and/or headache. Cervical vertigo can apparently be temporary or permanent.

The most common event putting all of this into motion is a whiplash accident or some other trauma involving the neck and head. And therein lies some of the problem for the theory of cervicogenic vertigo, when the neck is injured the head or inner ear may be injured as well. These vestibular symptoms could come from any of the three.

The diagnosis is usually made on the basis of the history and examination and the ruling out of any better explanations for the symptoms.

No objective test exists that can determine if symptoms are coming from the neck. No test can look at, or measure, the signals sent to the neck or those sent back up to the brain.

This is no magic bullet to make the symptoms go away—no surgery, no drugs. A combination of time, physical therapy for the neck and vestibular rehabilitation therapy are most commonly used. The prognosis is hard to predict with some cases being temporary and others lasting a very long time, possibly even permanently.

References and Reading List:

Brandt, T. "Cervical vertigo—reality or fiction?" *Audiology and Neurootology,* *1*(4):187-196, 1996.

Brandt, T., and Bronstein, A.M. "Cervical vertigo." *Journal of Neurology, Neurosurgery and Psychiatry, 71:8-12, 2001.*

Jongkees, L.B. "Cervical vertigo." *Laryngoscope, 79*(8):1473-1484, 1969.

Norre, M. E. "Neurophysiology of vertigo with special reference to cervical vertigo. A review." *Acta Belgica - Medica Physica, 9*(3):183-194, 1986.

Norre, M. E. "Cervical vertigo. Diagnostic and semiological problem with special emphasis upon "cervical nystagmus." *Acta Oto-Rhino-Laryngologica Belgica, 41*(3):436-452, 1987.

Vibert, D., Rohr-Le Floch, J., and Gauthier, G. "Vertigo as manifestation of vertebral artery dissection after chiropractic neck manipulations." *Journal of Otorhinolaryngology and It's Related Specialties,* 55:140-142, 1993.

Wrisley, D.M., Sparto, P.J., Whitney, S.L., and Furman, J.M. "Cervicogenic dizziness: a review of diagnosis and treatment." *Journal of Orthopedic Sports Physical Therapy,* 30(12):755-766, 2000.

Chapter Twenty
Cholesteatoma

A cholesteatoma is a cyst-like growth lined with cells just like those lining the middle ear and filled with keratin, a substance normally found in the hair and nails. They usually begin growing right on the inside of the eardrum but can be found throughout the temporal bone, the skull bone holding the inner ear. People are either born with it or develop it, usually after a long series of middle ear infections.

It's a disorder that can cause damage to the middle ear and surrounding areas, including the inner ear. When left alone cholesteatomas grow rapidly and cause bone destruction that can lead to hearing loss and possibly vestibular symptoms. Vestibular symptoms start if the cholesteatoma causes bone erosion and an abnormal opening called a perilymphatic fistula occurs allowing the inner ear fluids to leave the inner ear areas.

The vertigo caused by this damage is usually brought on or made worse by pressure changes such as sneezing, coughing, bearing down while on the toilet, and lifting heavy objects. It can occur at other times in other situations as well.

In most cases the diagnosis is based on the history and a look at the ear canal with a run-of-the-mill otoscope. A CT scan can also aid in making or confirming the diagnosis

Symptom blockers and avoidance of activities that bring on symptoms can help in the short term but the only effective treatment to stop the ongoing damage is surgery. The type surgery done will depend upon the location and size of the cholesteatoma and what damage it's already caused. Surgery ranges from simply removing the growth to total removal of most or all of the middle ear structures. Many surgeons will also do a follow-up endoscopy of the middle ear months after the surgery to see if the cholesteatoma has grown back.

If the vestibular damage is permanent and causing symptoms that decrease the quality of life or place a person at risk for accidents, other surgery aimed solely at the vertigo and vestibular symptoms may be suggested.

A textbook case of cholesteatoma would include:

- History of many middle ear infections
- Possibly ear drainage
- Presence of a hearing loss and perhaps vestibular problems
- Abnormal looking eardrum
- Abnormal imaging studies (CT, MRI or X-Rays)
- Dramatic symptom changes can occur during abrupt pressure changes

Cholesteatoma doesn't usually cause vestibular symptoms alone or out of the blue. The typical story is one of past middle ear infections and hearing loss.

References and Reading List:

Babighian, G. "Posterior and attic wall osteoplasty: hearing results and recurrence rates in cholesteatoma." *Otology and Neurotology*, 23(1):14-17, 2002.

Darrouzet, V., Duclos, J.Y., Portmann, D., and Bebear, J.P. "Congenital middle ear cholesteatomas in children: our experience in 34 cases." *Otolaryngology-Head and Neck Surgery*, 126(1):34-40, 2002.

Grayeli, A.B., Mosnier, I., El Garem, H., Bouccara, D., and Sterkers, O. "Extensive intratemporal cholesteatoma: surgical strategy." *American Journal of Otology*, 21(6):774-781, 2000.

Hasebe, S., Takahashi, H., Honjo, I., Miura, M., and Tanabe, M. "Mastoid condition and clinical course of cholesteatoma." *Journal of Otorhinolaryngology and It's Related Specialties*, 63(3):160-164, 2001.

Karmarkar, S., Bhatia, S., Saleh, E., DeDonato, G., Taibah, A., Russo, A., and Sanna, M. "Cholesteatoma surgery: the individualized technique." *Annals of Otology, Rhinology, and Laryngology*, 104(8):591-595, 1995.

Koltai, P.J., Nelson, M., Castellon, R.J., Garabedian, E.N., Triglia, J.M., Roman, S., and Roger, G. "The natural history of congenital cholesteatoma." *Archives of Otolaryngology-Head and Neck Surgery*, 128(7):804-809, 2002.

Lalwani, A.K., and Grundfast, K.M. *Pediatric otology and neurotology*. Philadelphia: Lippincott-Raven, 1998.

McKennanm, K.X. "Cholesteatoma: recognition and management." *American Family Physician*, 43(6):2091-2096, 1991.

Nelson, M., Roger, G., Koltai, P.J., Garabedian, E.N., Triglia, J.M., Roman, S., Castellon, R.J., and Hammel, J.P. "Congenital cholesteatoma: classification, management, and outcome." *Archives of Otolaryngology-Head and Neck Surgery*, 128(7):810-814, 2002.

Potsic, W.P., Korman, S.B., Samadi, D.S., and Wetmore, R.F. "Congenital cholesteatoma: 20 years' experience at The Children's Hospital of Philadelphia." *Otolaryngology-Head and Neck Surgery*, 126(4):409-414, 2002.

Robinson, J.M. "Cholesteatoma: skin in the wrong place." *Journal of the Royal Society of Medicine*, 90(2):93-96, 1997.

Sie, K.C. "Cholesteatoma in children." *Pediatric Clinics of North America*, 43(6):1245-1252, 1996.

Soldati, D., and Mudry, A. "Knowledge about cholesteatoma, from the first description to the modern histopathology." *Otology and Neurotology*, 22(6):723-730, 2001.

Tarabichi M. "Endoscopic management of cholesteatoma: long-term results." *Otolaryngology-Head and Neck Surgery,* 122(6):874-881, 2000.

Ueda, H., Nakashima, T., and Nakata, S. "Surgical strategy for cholesteatoma in children." *Auris Nasus Larynx,* 28(2):125-129, 2001.

Van den Abeele, D., and Offeciers, F.E. "Management of labyrinthine fistulas in cholesteatoma." *Acta Otorhinolaryngologica Belgique,* 47(3):311-321, 1993.

Yung, M.W. "The use of middle ear endoscopy: has residual cholesteatoma been eliminated?" *Journal of Laryngology and Otology,* 115(12):958-961, 2001.

Chapter Twenty-one
Delayed Endolymphatic Hydrops

In this uncommon disorder the amount of endolymph in one or both ears increases and the first symptom is separated from further symptoms by years.

There are two different "events" in this disorder, profound hearing loss or deafness in the normal ear of a child or young adult followed by problems in the same ear or the opposite ear years later. There are reports of the separation being as little as 6 years or as many as 50 years with the average around 16 years.

Two different versions exist, the same ear and the opposite ear types. When all the problems turn up in the same ear it's called ipsilateral delayed endolymphatic hydrops. It's contralateral endolymphatic hydrops if the first symptom is in one ear and the further symptoms occur in the opposite ear.

Same Ear

In this version of delayed endolymphatic hydrops profound hearing loss or deafness occur in the normal ear of a child or young adult. Years go by without any problems when suddenly attacks of vertigo, further hearing loss and tinnitus and/or ear fullness begin in the same ear. The symptoms can be identical to Meniere's disease with the history the only difference between them.

Other Ear

This variety differs a bit from the same ear type. Profound hearing loss or deafness occurs in the normal ear of a child or young adult. Years go by without any other ear problems when suddenly attacks of vertigo, hearing loss, and ear ringing and/or ear pressure begin in the opposite ear. The symptoms, again, are similar to Meniere's disease.

Nobody knows for sure why this disorder occurs in the first place let alone why it returns. One theory is that a virus attacks the ear, lives there quietly for years and then comes back to life for some unknown reason. Another theory is that the immune system goes haywire and starts attacking the ear, perhaps once early on and then again later. Another idea is that the initial hearing loss occurs for some reason, perhaps from a virus. The immune system then mistakenly identifies the ear as a foreign invader and attacks it later on.

The diagnosis of this disorder is based upon the history and hearing tests.

Unfortunately the treatments used by most doctors are no different than those used in the treatment of Meniere's disease and aren't as effective as anyone would like. Doctors viewing the disorder as an autoimmune reaction will treat it as such. They may also see hearing loss in the second ear as an emergency to be treated with steroids and other drugs capable of stopping the immune system attacks.

If deafness or profound hearing loss occurs in both ears a cochlear implant can be effective in bringing back a degree of sound.

The prognosis is hard to predict but people with both ears affected can end up with a severe hearing disability that may be more of a burden than the vestibular symptoms.

References and Reading List:

Aso, S., and Watanabe, Y. "Electrocochleography in the diagnosis of delayed endolymphatic hydrops." *Acta Otolaryngologica,* Supplement 511:87-90, 1994.

Harcourt, J.P., and Brookes, G.B. "Delayed endolymphatic hydrops: clinical manifestations and treatment outcome." *Clinical Otolaryngology,* 20(4):318-322, 1995.

Harris, J.P., and Aframian, D. "Role of autoimmunity in contralateral delayed endolymphatic hydrops." *American Journal of Otology,* 15(6):710-716, 1994.

Hashimoto, S., Furukawa, K., and Sasaki, T. "Treatment of ipsilateral delayed endolymphatic hydrops." *Acta Otolaryngologica,* Supplement 528:113-15, 1997.

Hicks, G.W., and Wright, J.W. "Delayed endolymphatic hydrops: a review of 15 cases." *Laryngoscope,* 98(8 Pt 1):840-845, 1988.

Huang, T.S., and Lin, C.C. "Delayed endolymphatic hydrops: study and review of clinical implications and surgical treatment." *Ear Nose Throat Journal,* 80(2):76-78, 81-82, 84 passim, 2001.

Kumagami, H., and Sasano, T. "A case of delayed endolymphatic hydrops." *Auris Nasus Larynx,* 19(1):51-54, 1992.

Lambert, P.R. "Delayed vertigo and profound sensorineural hearing loss." *Laryngoscope,* 95(12):1541-1544, 1985.

LeLiever, W.C., and Barber, H.O. "Delayed endolymphatic hydrops." *Journal of Otolaryngology,* 9(5):375-380, 1980.

Nadol, J.B., Weiss, A.D., and Parker, S.W. "Vertigo of delayed onset after sudden deafness." *Annals of Otology, Rhinology, and Laryngology,* 84(6):841-846, 1975.

Ohki, M., Matsuzaki, M., Sugasawa, K., and Murofushi, T. "Vestibular evoked myogenic potentials in patients with contralateral delayed endolymphatic hydrops." *European Archives of Otorhinolaryngology,* 259(1):24-26, 2002.

Schuknecht, H.F., Suzuka, Y., and Zimmermann, C. "Delayed endolymphatic hydrops and its relationship to Meniere's disease." *Annals of Otology, Rhinology, and Laryngology,* 99(11):843-853, 1990.

Shojaku, H., Takemori, S., Kobayashi, K., and Watanabe, Y. "Clinical usefulness of glycerol vestibular-evoked myogenic potentials: preliminary report." *Acta Otolaryngologica*, Supplement 545:65-68, 2001.

Yaku, Y., and Komatsuzaki, A. "Ultrastructure of the vestibular sensory organs in delayed endolymphatic hydrops." *American Journal of Otolaryngology*, 10(5):336-341, 1989.

Yazdi, A.K., and Rutka, J. "Results of labyrinthectomy in the treatment of Meniere's disease and delayed endolymphatic hydrops." *Journal of Otolaryngology*, 25(1):26-31, 1996.

Chapter Twenty-two
Endolymphatic Hydrops

Technically endolymphatic hydrops means an increased amount of endolymph in the inner ear. Nothing complicated about that, right? Well unfortunately it isn't as clear-cut as it sounds because the term endolymphatic hydrops can be used in a number of different ways. It can refer to a physical change within the inner ear, a specific disorder or a group of disorders.

Physical Change
Endolymphatic hydrops means too much endolymph. Because the inner ear is encased in bone, an increase in the fluids within it can cause the membranes to rupture and the cells to be squished. Both the increase in fluid and the damage it causes are called endolymphatic hydrops

Endolymphatic hydrops can only be seen and measured with precision after life. There is one test for endolymphatic hydrops, the electrocochleogram or ECOG. Unfortunately the test can also be positive in normal people and negative in people with symptoms making it a lot less dependable than a direct pressure measurement or a picture of the inside of the inner would be, if they existed. Some experts feel the test only points to a fluid problem within the inner ear and not which one.

Specific Disorder
The term endolymphatic hydrops is also used to refer to a specific disorder like delayed endolymphatic hydrops, idiopathic endolymphatic hydrops, or secondary endolymphatic hydrops

This isn't as neat and organized as it sounds. Technically Meniere's disease is defined by the Committee on Hearing and Equilibrium of the American Academy of Otolaryngology-Head and Neck Surgery as idiopathic endolymphatic hydrops. Some doctors drop off the word idiopathic and just refer to it as endolymphatic hydrops. The international organization assigning numbers to all diseases and disorders of the body have given the same number to Meniere's disease and endolymphatic hydrops making matters even worse.

When a doctor feels a person's symptoms are from increased endolymph but the symptoms don't fit the criteria for Meniere's disease they may simply call it endolymphatic hydrops.

Group of Disorders
Lastly, the term endolymphatic hydrops can be used to refer to a group of conditions that

include Meniere's disease, secondary endolymphatic hydrops, and delayed endolymphatic hydrops.

Meniere's disease is a disorder of unknown cause in which there are attacks of vertigo, hearing loss and ear ringing or ear fullness.

Secondary endolymphatic hydrops is endolymphatic hydrops occurring as the result of another condition such as allergy, middle ear infection, syphilis or a head injury.

Delayed endolymphatic hydrops is a disorder in which deafness or hearing loss occurs in an otherwise normal ear early in life followed years late by episodic vertigo in the same ear or the opposite ear.

Reference:

"Committee on Hearing and Equilibrium guidelines for the diagnosis and evaluation of therapy in Meniere's disease." American Academy of Otolaryngology-Head and Neck Foundation, Inc., *Otolaryngology-Head and Neck Surgery,* 113(3):181-5, 1995.

Chapter Twenty-three
Enlarged Vestibular Aqueduct Syndrome

The vestibular aqueduct is a tunnel running from the vestibule of the inner ear through the temporal bone toward the brain. It contains the endolymphatic duct and the endolymphatic sac along with an artery and vein.

Sometimes, for an unknown reason, the aqueduct stops developing during the fifth week of fetal growth before the usual narrowing has occurred leaving it wider than normal. Once the bone surrounding the aqueduct hardens the wide shape is permanent.

When a person has a hearing loss, possibly vestibular symptoms, along with an aqueduct larger than 1.5mm, they are said to have enlarged vestibular aqueduct syndrome or large vestibular aqueduct syndrome.

The hearing loss can come on suddenly and massively, be lost bit-by-bit over time, or come and go over time. Vestibular symptoms can occur but the current wisdom is that they aren't very frequent and when they do occur they're mild. It's possible to have an enlarged aqueduct and experience only vestibular symptoms but that's out of the ordinary.

One group of doctors in Turkey reported that vestibular symptoms could include vertigo after looking at revolving objects, spontaneous episodes of vertigo and/or a more or less constant sort of dizziness.

Symptoms may first be noticed after head trauma, diving into water, scuba diving or an upper respiratory infection like a cold. Someone with this disorder is usually told to avoid head trauma, diving, scuba diving and upper respiratory infections and the like because they can worsen the condition at any time. In children this means no contact sports.

This problem can only be diagnosed with a CT scan. As many as 60% of people with this disorder also have other bony abnormalities that themselves can cause hearing loss and vestibular problems.

Unfortunately with the current state of technology an enlarged aqueduct can't be fixed. A hearing aid may help with the hearing loss and further hearing loss may be limited by avoiding head trauma and upper respiratory infections.

Because the cause of vestibular symptoms isn't understood, treatment options are limited to grin and bare it or trying to cover up the symptoms with drugs. Surgery has been tried on some folks but without any improvement in hearing—current wisdom is that surgery doesn't help.

There really is no typical case of enlarged vestibular aqueduct syndrome making accurate predictions of the future impossible.

References and Reading List:

Arcand, P., Desrosiers, M., Dube, J., and Abela, A. "The large vestibular aqueduct syndrome and sensorineural hearing loss in the pediatric population." *Journal of Otolaryngology*, 20:247-250, 1991.

Bent, J.P., Chute, P., and Parisier, S.C. "Cochlear implantation in children with enlarged vestibular aqueducts." *Laryngoscope*, 109:1019-1022, 1999.

Emmett, J.R. "The large vestibular aqueduct syndrome." *American Journal of Otology*, 6:387-403, 1985.

Go, E., Shim, W., Roh, H., Wang, S., and Chon, K. "Familial enlarged vestibular aqueduct syndrome." *American Journal of Otolaryngology*, 22:286-290, 2001.

Harker, L.A., Vanderheiden, S., Veazey, D., Gentile, N., and McCleary, E. "Multichannel cochlear implantation in children with large vestibular aqueduct syndrome." *Annals of Otology, Rhinology, and Laryngology*, Supplement 177:39-43, 1999.

Jackler, R.K., and De La Cruz, A. "The large vestibular aqueduct syndrome." *Laryngoscope*, 99:1238-1243, 1989.

Levenson, M.J., Parisier, S.C., Jacobs, M., and Edelstein, D.R. "The large vestibular aqueduct syndrome in children." *Archives of Otolaryngology-Head and Neck Surgery*, 115:54-58, 1989.

Manolis, E.N., Eavey, R.D., Cunningham, M.J., and Weber, A.L. "Enlarged vestibular aqueduct as a marker for hearing loss in children." *Clinical Pediatrics*, 37:689-692, 1998.

Oh, A.K., Ishiyama, A., and Baloh, R.W. "Vertigo and the enlarged vestibular aqueduct syndrome." *Journal of Neurology*, 248(11):971-974, 2001.

Phelps, P.S. "Large vestibular aqueduct: large endolymphatic sac?" *Journal of Laryngology and Otology*, 110:1103-1104, 1996.

Reussner, L.A., Dutcher, P., and House, W.F. "Large vestibular aqueduct syndrome with massive endolymphatic sacs." *Otolaryngology-Head and Neck Surgery*, 113:606-610, 1995.

Schessel, D.A., and Nedzelski, J.M. "Presentation of large vestibular aqueduct syndrome to a dizziness unit." *Journal of Otolaryngology-Head and Neck Surgery*, 21:265-269, 1992.

Usami, S., Abe, S., Weston, M.D., Shinkawa, H., Van Camp, G., and Kinberling, W.J. "Non-syndromic hearing loss associated with enlarged vestibular aqueduct is caused by PDS mutations." *Human Genetics*, 104:188-192, 1999.

Valvassori, G.E. "The large vestibular aqueduct and associated anomalies of the inner ear." *Otolaryngologic Clinics of North America*, 16:95-101, 1983.

Valvassori, G.E., and Clemis, J.D. "The large vestibular aqueduct syndrome." *Laryngoscope*, 88:723-728, 1978.

Welling, D.B., Martyn, M.D., Miles, B.A., Oehler, M., and Schmalbrock, P. "Endolymphatic sac occlusion for the enlarged vestibular aqueduct syndrome." *American Journal of Otology*, 19:145-151, 1998.

Welling, D.B., Slater, P.W., Martyn, M.D., Antonelli, P.J., Gantz, B.J., Luxford, W.M., and Shelton, C. "Sensorineural hearing loss after occlusion of the enlarged vestibular aqueduct." *American Journal of Otology*, 20:338-343, 1999.

Yetiser, S., Kertmen, M., and Ozkaptan, Y. "Vestibular disturbances in patients with large vestibular aqueduct syndrome (LVAS)." *Acta Otolaryngologica*, 119:641-646, 1999.

Chapter Twenty-four
Immune System Diseases

Along with everything else bad that can happen, the inner ear can also fall victim to an immune system gone haywire. (Otherwise known as an autoimmune disorder or reaction in which the immune system, for some reason, identifies the body as a foreign invader and attacks it. In some ways this is similar to what happens when the body rejects or attacks a transplanted organ). In some autoimmune disorders a small area of the body is attacked, in others the attack affects large areas, sometimes the entire body. Of all the people with autoimmune disorders 2/3 are woman and most are in the 20 to 50 year old age group.

The inner ear can apparently be the only target of the immune system run amok or it can be one of many areas targeted for retribution. Debris from a distant attack may also be able to float through the blood stream into the inner ear and cause problems.

Autoimmune inner ear disorders have their troubles and controversies: They're based a bit more on ideas, theories and comparisons to other body systems then on hard, physical evidence within the inner ear; they're tough to recognize; within specialized medicine they belong more to the rheumatologist, then to the otolaryngologist (ENT); some doctors feel these disorders should be called immune mediated inner ear disorders instead and some have other names for them; in the minds of many ENT's they cause hearing loss, not vestibular symptoms and an autoimmune diagnosis as an explanation for vestibular symptoms is rarely made.

Unfortunately it's easier to diagnose one of these conditions after the damage is severe and possibly permanent. Why? It looks like a lot of other inner ear disorders and doesn't seem special until the hearing loss is massive and/or the other ear is rapidly involved.

Although there are blood tests, many are expensive, take a long time to conduct, may be sent away, they are outside an ENT's usual area of expertise and tests can be positive when the illness isn't present and negative when it is—they aren't always as much help as anyone would like.

As a consequence a doctor is left at times depending upon their own experience and textbook descriptions of histories and symptoms to make the diagnosis.

Disorders
Inner ear alone
Autoimmune inner ear disease (AIED), the autoimmune problem involving only the inner ear, was first identified and written about in 1979. It consists of massive hearing loss in one ear followed in weeks to months by the other ear, resulting in total or near total deafness. Symptoms can fluctuate a bit but the more usual story is one of a downward spiral. Hearing loss is usually

considered to be THE symptom in this disorder but vestibular symptoms may be present in as many as 50%.

Steroids usually help people with AIED. This steroid "responsiveness" is now used by some doctors to help make the diagnosis. If high dose steroids given for a week or two improve things it's thought the problem might be autoimmune and more steroids, or other drugs, are used to treat it. If high dose steroids over a week or two don't help it's assumed an autoimmune reaction isn't the problem.

Blood tests might also be done to help make the diagnosis. There are general blood tests like the eosinophil sedimentation rate (sometimes called a sed rate) that can only show a problem of some sort, some place in the body but not what type or where. There are also other tests like the lymphocyte transformation test and the test for anticochlear antibodies that may give a bit more specific information.

There are also similar reports of massive vestibular losses in both ears occurring rapidly in a few people. It's not known if they are having a vestibular version of AIED.

Inner ears and eyes
In 1945 Cogan's Syndrome, involving both the eyes and ears, was first described in a medical journal. In this disorder a number of symptoms including episodes of vertigo, hearing loss, ear ringing and red painful eyes begin over a short period of time, usually 1 to 24 months.

The most common cause of these painful red eyes is interstitial keratitis but some experts feel episcleritis, scleritis or choroiditis may also occur in Cogan's.

This is a rare condition with few studies available but there are some published statistics:

- 6% are blind within 2 years
- 43-95% have massive hearing loss
- 71% have symptoms beyond the eyes and ears such as anemia, weight loss, fever, arthritis, gastrointestinal dysfunction, enlarged lymph nodes, enlarged spleen, cerebral artery occlusion, aortic insufficiency (10%)

There must be evidence of inner ear, eye and autoimmune involvement for this diagnosis to be made. Cogan's is particularly difficult to diagnose because it requires teamwork between an ENT, ophthalmologist and a rheumatologist (autoimmune disorder expert). Unfortunately no medical specialty covers the eye, ears and autoimmune disorders as one package.

In addition, getting in for an eye examination when the eyes are red and inflamed is crucial but very tough. If your eyes don't act up for a scheduled doctors appointment get your ophthalmologist to agree to see you in the office any time they are acting up. You can also ask that they see you in their hospitals' ER if your eye symptoms flare up on a weekend when their office isn't open. If this isn't possible have a camera set to go and photograph or videotape your eyes so your doctor can see what you're talking about.

Miscellaneous
Inner ear symptoms can also occur from a body wide autoimmune disorder like systemic lupus erythematosus, Wegener's granulomatosus, vasculitits, ulcerative colitis, rheumatoid arthritis, thyroid disorders, relapsing polychondritis, polyarteritis nodosa, and/or Sjögren s syndrome.

Neither an ENT nor a rheumatologist is trained to do a complete eye examination. An ophthalmologist and rheumatologist can't evaluate inner ear balance. The ENT and ophthalmologist aren't in the best position to diagnose and treat autoimmune disorders.

They have to work together for a person to receive the most knowledgeable care and advice. Unfortunately many people don't have access to such a team.

In general, it seems that hearing loss is more likely to occur but vestibular symptoms are quite possible. The symptoms can fluctuate or just get worse and worse.

The diagnosis of a vestibular problem secondary to an autoimmune problem is tricky because it just isn't possible to know with scientific certainty if the inner ear symptoms and/or damage are from the body-wide autoimmune problem or if an inner ear problem is occurring all on it's own. The diagnosis is really an educated guess.

Treatment
The treatment depends upon the disorder, the symptoms, the damage, the individual with it and the prior experience and knowledge of the doctor.

The cause should be treated when possible. In autoimmune problems this is done with drugs that can slow down or stop the immune system from its attack. There are a handful of drugs that can be used: steroids, methotrexate, Enbrel (etanercept) and cyclophosphomide. All are given by pill or injection for months, possibly even years, not for days. You must be committed to taking these drugs properly and watching for any side effects and problems such as the increased tendency to develop infections.

Another approach is the injection of steroids directly into the ear. The major drawback with this treatment: it can't treat a body-wide or distant autoimmune disorder.

Steroid eye drops may also be used in the case of Cogan's syndrome. These will only help the eyes; they can't stop the underlying problem or help the ears.

On occasion a doctor may prescribe plasmaphoresis to remove substances from the blood stream. It's done in a way that's similar to dialysis with blood removed, filtered and returned to the body. If this treatment is recommended check and double check with your insurance company about your coverage. Some companies consider this treatment to be experimental or unproven for inner ear symptoms and may refuse payment. The most frequent criticism of the treatment is that any positive effects are short lived so it isn't worth the expense and risk of the treatment.

In addition to going after the underlying problem, treatments aimed at the physical changes caused by the diseases can be used as well. For example, endolymphatic hydrops may be the end result of an autoimmune disorder in some people. When that's the case a low salt diet and/or diuretics may be of help.

If the hearing loss progresses to deafness in both ears a cochlear implant can be used, which is exactly what happened to Rush Limbaugh in the summer of 2001.

Prognosis
This varies—a lot. In a few people the symptoms are stopped and the damage undone by aggressive treatment. Others have a reduction in symptoms and no further damage. Unfortunately the disease process may also go on unchecked.

References and Reading List:
Bernstein, J.M., Shanahan, T.C., and Schaffer, F.M. "Further observations on the role of the MHC genes and certain hearing disorders." *Acta Otolaryngologica,* 116(5):666-671, 1996.

Berrocal, J.R., Ramirez-Camacho, R., Vargas, J.A., and Millan, I. "Does the serological testing really play a role in the diagnosis of immune-mediated inner ear disease?" *Acta Otolaryngologica,* 122:243-248, 2002.

Campbell, K.C., and Klemens, J.J. "Sudden hearing loss and autoimmune inner ear disease." *Journal of the American Academy of Audiology*, 11(7):361-367, 2000.

Hirose, K., Wener, M.H., and Duckert, L.G. "Utility of laboratory testing in autoimmune inner ear disease." *Laryngoscope*, 109(11):1749-1754, 1999.

Lasak, J.M., Sataloff, R.T., Hawkshaw, M., Carey, T.E., Lyons, K.M., and Spiegel, J.R. "Autoimmune inner ear disease: steroid and cytotoxic drug therapy." *Ear Nose Throat Journal*, 80(11):808-11, 815-816, 818, 2001.

Luetje, C.M., and Berliner, K.I. "Plasmaphereis in autoimmune inner ear disease: long-term follow-up." *American Journal of Otology*, 18:572-576, 1997.

McCabe, B. "Autoimmune sensorineural hearing loss." *Annals of Otolaryngology*, 88:585-589, 1979.

Pollak, L., Luxon, L.M., and Haskard, D.O. "Labyrinthine involvement in Behcet's syndrome." *Journal of Laryngology and Otology*, 115: 522-529, 2001.

Rahman, M.U., Poe, D.S., and Choi, H.K. "Etanercept therapy for immune-mediated cochleovestibular disorders: preliminary results in a pilot study." *Otology and Neurotology*, 22:619-624, 2001.

Roland, J.T. "Autoimmune inner ear disease." *Current Rheumatology Reports*, 2(2):171-174, 2000.

Sismanis, A., Wise, C.M., and Johnson, G.D. "Methotrexate management of immune-mediated cochleovestibular disorders." *Otolaryngology-Head and Neck Surgery*, 116:146-152, 1997.

Stone, J. H., and Francis, H.W. "Immune-mediated inner ear disease." *Current Opinions in Rheumatology*, 12:32-40, 2000.

Tumiati, B., and Casoli, P. "Sudden sensorineural hearing loss and anticardiolipin antibody." *American Journal of Otolaryngology*, 16(3):220, 1995.

Yang, G.S., Song, H.T., Keithley, E.M., and Harris, J.P. "Intratympanic immunosuppressives for prevention of immune-mediated sensorineural hearing loss." *American Journal of Otology*, 21(4):499-504, 2000.

Yeo, S.W. and Park, S.N. "Immune-mediated sensorineural hearing loss in a patient with ankylosing spondylitis: a case report." *Otolaryngology-Head and Neck Surgery*, 125:113-114, 2001.

Chapter Twenty-five
Labyrinthitis

Labyrinthitis is an inflammation of the inner ear. Labyrinth is another name for the inner ear and the suffix -itis means inflammation. There are several types of labyrinthitis including viral, bacterial and serous (that's serous, not serious).

Viral Labyrinthitis

This is an inflammation of the inner ear areas caused by a virus. In some cases the virus causing the problem is known because it's infecting other body areas as well which is the case with both the cytomegalovirus and the mumps viruses.

In most cases the virus isn't identified and only seems to affect the inner ear, causing both vestibular and hearing symptoms. The symptoms begin suddenly in one ear and include hearing loss, tinnitus and vertigo. It can be the sort of vertigo that causes a person to lie on their side in bed hanging on to their pillow with one hand and something to vomit into with the other. Although it probably feels like forever the vertigo does begin to stop in 24 to 48 hours. It can be another 5 days before a person can get up and move about on their own. At first they'll have trouble walking in a straight line and probably lean to the side and have motion insensitivity. It can be as many as 6 weeks before they feel fit enough to go back to work. Feelings of imbalance last as long as 6 months after the episode in some people.

The vertigo is bad because the flow of information from the inner ear to the brain is cut off abruptly. If this damage is permanent the other ear should be able to take over in the following weeks through vestibular compensation. Anti-vomiting and anti-vestibular drugs should be stopped as early as possible during the illness because they might slow this process down.

This diagnosis is an assumption because there's no way, in a living person, to prove that the inner ear is under attack from a virus. Removal of inner ear fluids for viral testing isn't done because it would cause more damage than the disease itself. An MRI may show an inner ear change but can't prove if a virus is the culprit. Some vestibular tests will also show an abnormality but not if a virus is at fault. A blood test can be done to look for a body wide viral problem such as the cytomegalovirus but a positive result doesn't prove the virus is causing the problem within the ear.

In the majority of cases the virus isn't known but some experts feel it could very well be the herpes simplex virus I (HSV-I) causing the problem. Researchers, under very special research conditions, have found this virus in the inner ears of a few people.

Because there aren't good tests for this disorder the diagnosis is based on the history and examination along with a hearing test.

Treatments that can be used include:

- Grin and bear it
- Suppress the symptoms
- Anti-inflammatory drugs such as steroids
- Anti-viral drugs
- IV fluids if vomiting is uncontrollable

Since it can't be determined with scientific certainty if labyrinthitis and vestibular neuronitis are separate disorders some doctors lump them together.

Bacterial Labyrinthitis
Bacterial labyrinthitis is an inflammation and infection of the inner ear caused by bacteria. It's also called suppurative labyrinthitis. This doesn't come out of the blue or alone. It develops from meningitis or a middle ear infection or as a nasty complication of ear surgery.

The symptoms are similar to the viral type but also include those of meningitis or a middle ear infection. These include fever, rigid neck, visual light insensitivity, headache, ear drainage, pain, swelling or redness in or around the ear and a general feeling of being very ill. Unlike the viral variety this one can affect both ears and the inner ear damage can be both extensive and permanent.

It's diagnosed with the history and examination and the presence of meningitis or a middle ear infection.

The treatment includes antibiotics to treat both the underlying infection and the infected inner ear, anti-vomiting drugs, anti-vertigo drugs, and IV fluids/hospital care if need be.

Serous Labyrinthitis
This inflammation occurs when problem substances from the middle ear pass through the membrane covered openings into the inner ear. It is the most common complication of a middle ear infection. Serous labyrinthitis is also called toxic labyrinthitis (but has nothing to do with the vestibular disorder ototoxicity).

The inner ear symptoms include hearing loss, tinnitus and vestibular symptoms ranging from minor imbalance to the sort of vertigo that puts people to bed for a day or two. Symptoms of middle ear infection (otitis media) include ear pain, warmth, swelling, fever, hearing loss, and drainage that might have pus in it.

Again there is no X-Ray, blood test, etc. that can diagnose this problem. The diagnosis is based upon the history and examination.

The treatment is aimed first at the cause. In the case of a middle ear infection antibiotics are given and a small incision might be made through the eardrum. Drugs to help with the vomiting, nausea and vertigo are given as needed.

References and Reading List:
Arbusow, V., Theil, D., Strupp, M., Mascolo, A., and Brandt. T. "HSV-1 is not only in human vestibular ganglia but also in the vestibular labyrinth." *Audiology and Neurootology*, 6(5):259-262, 2001.

Davis, L.E. "Viruses and vestibular neuritis: review of human and animal studies" *Acta Otolaryngologica*, Supplement 503:70-73, 1993.

Davis, L.E., and Johnsson, L.G. "Viral infections of the inner ear: clinical, virologic, and pathologic studies in humans and animals." *American Journal of Otolaryngology*, 4(5):347-362, 1983.

Hyden, D. "Mumps labyrinthitis, endolymphatic hydrops and sudden deafness in succession in the same ear.*" Journal of Otorhinolaryngology*, 58(6):338-342, 1996.

Kumagami, H. "Detection of viral antigen in the endolymphatic sac." *European Archives of Otorhinolaryngology*, 253(4-5):264-267, 1996.

Mafee, M.F. "MR imaging of intralabyrinthine schwannoma, labyrinthitis, and other labyrinthine pathology." *American Journal of Otolaryngology*, 11(6):382-388, 1990.

Nomura, Y., Harada, T., and Hara, M. "Viral infection and the inner ear." *Journal of Otorhinolaryngology and Related Specialties*, 50(4):201-211, 1988.

Savitt, L.E. "Intermittent herpes simplex.*" Archives of Otolaryngology-Head and Neck Surgery*, 115(2):248, 1989.

Chapter Twenty-six
Lyme Disease

Lyme disease is an infection spread by the bite of a tick that can have body wide affects, some of them quite serious. It occurs throughout areas of the U.S., Europe and Asia.

Technical point: Lyme disease is caused by the spirochete borrelia burgdorferi.

During the early stage, in the weeks after a bite, about 80% of people develop a rash that spreads around the body. Many also develop flu-like symptoms including malaise (that tired, unmotivated, don't want to be bothered, don't care, sick feeling that accompanies many illnesses), fatigue, headache, joint pain, muscle pain, fever, and swollen lymph nodes.

If untreated the disease can move on to affect the central nervous system or brain in 5 to 15% of people. Serious illnesses like meningitis (inflammation of the coverings of the brain) or encephalitis (inflammation of the brain itself) can occur at this time as well as inflammation of the optic nerve (vision nerve) or facial nerve (facial muscle movement nerve) and maybe the vestibular branch of the vestibulocochlear nerve.

Lyme disease is known to be capable of causing facial muscle paralysis. Since the facial nerve travels with the vestibulocochlear nerve from the brain to the ear it isn't hard to imagine the disease might also be capable of infecting the vestibulocochlear nerve.

It's pretty hard to know how big a vestibular problem Lyme disease is. Some Lyme disease experts feel vestibular symptoms can be a part of the disorder, while others don't feel that way. In one Finnish study everyone seen in an ENT a clinic with vestibular symptoms between 1987 and 1990 was tested for Lyme. Of the 350 people in the study 12 had positive Lyme disease blood tests. Still, many general ENT's may never think about Lyme as a cause of vestibular symptoms.

The vestibular symptoms and problems Lyme might cause have not been researched very well. In one study of 266 people with Lyme disease 25.9% had "dizziness," 5.3% ear pain, 5% tinnitus, 4.1% fullness and 1.4% had hearing loss from both ears. They also found that some people had spinning vertigo coming in episodes, others positional vertigo and still others had a symptom pattern similar to vestibular neuritis.

The chance of a person having Lyme disease when they are experiencing inner ear symptoms alone, is pretty remote. But, if someone already has Lyme disease and then develops vestibular symptoms there's a realistic chance Lyme disease is the cause.

Lyme is diagnosed by the history, the likelihood of having had a run-in with a tick, physical signs, symptoms and blood tests. Blood tests look for the body's response to Lyme disease and not for the bug itself. As a result the disease can be present even if the blood tests are negative and a blood test can be positive under certain conditions when the disease isn't present.

There is no test that can prove with scientific certainty that the cause of a person's vestibular disorder is Lyme. Blood tests, to some degree, can show if Lyme is affecting the body and vestibular tests can show, at times, if there is a vestibular problem in general, but no test can put the two together for sure.

If Lyme disease is suspected, antibiotic treatment based on the Centers for Disease Control guidelines can be started and if there's an improvement in all symptoms, including the vestibular ones, it can be concluded that the problem was Lyme.

If you have this disorder or think you might, there are several organizations you can get information and moral support from:

Lyme Disease Resource Center
PO Box 707
Weaverville, CA 96093
www.lymedisease.org

Lyme Disease Foundation
One Financial Plaza, 18th Floor
Hartford, CT 06103
www.lyme.org

The Lyme Disease Network
www.lymenet.org

References and Reading List:

Goldfarb, D., and Sataloff, R.T. "Lyme disease: a review for the otolaryngologist." *Ear Nose Throat Journal*, 73(11):824-829, 1994.

Heininger, U., Ries, M., Christ, P., and Harms, D. "Simultaneous palsy of facial and vestibular nerve in a child with Lyme borreliosis." *European Journal of Pediatrics*, 149(11):781-782, 1990.

Hyden, D., Roberg, M., and Odkvist, L. "Borreliosis as a cause of sudden deafness and vestibular neuritis in Sweden." *Acta Otolaryngologica*, Supplement 520 Pt 2:320-322, 1995.

Ishizaki, H., Pyykko, I., and Nozue, M. "Neuroborreliosis in the etiology of vestibular neuronitis." *Acta Otolaryngologica*, Supplement 503:67-69, 1993.

Moscatello, A.L., Worden, D.L., Nadelman, R.B., Wormser, G., and Lucente, F. "Otolaryngologic aspects of Lyme disease." *Laryngoscope*, 101(6 Pt 1):592-595, 1991.

Nields, J.A., Fallon, B.A., and Jastreboff, P.J. "Carbamazepine in the treatment of Lyme disease-induced hyperacusis." *Journal of Neuropsychiatry and Clinical Neurosciences*, 11(1):97-99, 1999.

Nields, J.A., and Kueton, J.F. "Tullio phenomenon and seronegative lyme borreliosis." *The Lancet*, 338(8759):128-129, 1991.

Peltomaa, M., Pyykko, I., Seppala, I., and Viljanen, M. "Lyme borreliosis—an unusual cause of vertigo." *Auris Nasus Larynx*, 25(3):233-242, 1998.

Selmani, Z., Pyykko, I., Ishizaki, H., and Ashammakhi, N. "Use of electrocochleography for assessing endolymphatic hydrops in patients with Lyme disease and Meniere's disease." *Acta Otolaryngologica*, 122(2):173-178, 2002.

Steere, A.C. "Lyme Disease." *New England Journal of Medicine*, 345(2):115-123, 2001.

Chapter Twenty-seven
Mal de Debarquement

If you've ever gone on a cruise and felt like you were still moving once back on terra firma you've felt the prominent symptom of this disorder.

Mal de Debarquement literally means sickness of disembarkment. Originally this referred only to movement symptoms developing right after ocean travel but now planes, trains and other movement are also included. Some doctors may also call it Mal de Debarquement syndrome or persistent mal de debarquement.

There isn't much about this disorder that's clear including its definition. At what point does a normal post-cruise movement sensation become mal de debarquement the disorder? How long after the cruise can the symptoms begin? There's no official answer to these questions, each doctor, including those studying and writing about the disorder, decides on their own.

Rocking, rolling, boat like movements or a sensation like floating in the ocean are common descriptions of the movement. All of these can be classified as vertigo since they are a sensation of movement that isn't occurring. A feeling of unsteadiness may also be present. The strength of the symptoms and the difficulties they bring on can vary a lot, from a minor inconvenience to incapacitation.

The following ARE NOT a part of mal de debarquement: Hearing loss, tinnitus, ear pressure/fullness, or episodes of strong rotational vertigo with nausea and/or vomiting.

Some people find relief from the rocking and other movement while walking or riding in a car. On the flip side the intensity may increase when still, like when in bed trying to fall asleep.

Unfortunately the diagnosis is not made very often and most information about the disorder has come from casual observation, not rigorous scientific inquiry. There are huge gaps in what we know about it. The only thing that's known for sure is that it exists but what it is and how to deal with it are pretty murky areas.

So What is it and Where Does it Come From?

It's pretty unlikely that taking a cruise or riding in a train can cause inner ear or nerve damage. That puts the spotlight on the brain and how it processes movement information. One educated guess is that in order to move about on a ship the brain becomes accustomed to sending repetitive muscle movement signals. Once back on land the same signals continue to be sent but are now wrong for the situation, causing a rocking sensation.

Another guess is that movement on a ship or train causes a nearly constant mismatch between visual and vestibular information sent to the brain. The eyes say a person is not moving in relation to their surroundings and the vestibular information says they are. The brain gets used to the mismatch and is able to ignore or override it. Once the cruise is done the mismatch between visual and vestibular information also stops but the brain doesn't realize this and a rocking sensation is the result.

Mal de Debarquement is defined by a symptom because there is no physical change, or at least nobody has stumbled into one yet. There is no specific test to detect this disorder. Instead tests are done in an attempt to figure out what isn't wrong. If nothing else can be found and the symptoms started after a cruise or other method of travel then the diagnosis of Mal de Debarquement may be made.

Not only is there no specific test, there's also no specific, generally accepted treatment for this disorder. Many treatments are available but whether or not one will help an individual can only be determined through trial and error.

Some treatments offered include:

- Walking outdoors looking at the horizon
- Drugs of the benzodiazepine family such as Klonopin and Valium
- Anti-motion sickness drugs like meclizine
- Anti-depressant drugs
- Vestibular Rehabilitation Therapy

Luckily in many people it just goes away as mysteriously as it appeared, with or without treatment.

This is a very difficult disorder to deal with because so little is really known about it. Without a physical change to look for, Mal de Debarquement is difficult to diagnose. If it can't be diagnosed with certainty trying to study any aspect of it is difficult because it's impossible to know if everyone in the study really had it. Another problem is that people who have never been on a cruise or ridden in a train or airplane can develop the same symptom. Do they have the same disorder or is it different in someway? Should they be treated and studied in the same way? To top this all off very few general doctors have heard about the disorder and some may even think it's a psychological problem rather than a physical ailment.

If you have this disorder or think you might, there are two internet organizations you can get information and moral support from: The Mal de Debarquement Syndrome web page at www.etete.com/mdd/ and the MdDS Balance Disorder Foundation site at www.nhffoundations.net/synapse/homepage/view.cfm?Edit_id=45&website=nhffoundations.net/MdDS

References and Reading List:
Baloh, R.W. *Dizziness, hearing loss, and tinnitus.* Philadelphia: F.A. Davis Company, 1998.

Baloh, R.W., and Halmagi, G.M. *Disorders of the vestibular system.* New York: Oxford University Press, 1996.

Brown, J.J., and Baloh, R.W. "Persistent Mal de Debarquement syndrome: a motion-induced subjective disorder of balance." *American Journal of Otolarynoglogy,* 8(4):219-222, 1987.

Cohen, H. "Vertigo after sailing a nineteenth century ship." *Journal of Vestibular Research,* 6(1):31-35, 1996.

Cohen, H. "Mild Mal de DeBarquement after sailing." *Annals of the New York Academy of Sciences,* 781:598-600, 1996.

Gordon, C.R., Spitzer, O., Shupak, A., and Doweck, I. "Survey of Mal de Debarquement." *British Medical Journal, 304*(6826):544, 1992.

Gordon, C.R., Spitzer, O., Doweck, I., Melamed, Y., and Shupak, A. "Clinical features of Mal De Debarquement: adaptation and habituation to sea conditions." *Journal of Vestibular Research,* 5(5):363-369, 1995.

Gordon, C.R., Shupak, A., and Nachum, Z. "Mal de DeBarquement," *Archives of Otolaryngology-Head and Neck Surgery, 126*(6):805-806, 2000.

Hain, T.C., Hanna, P.A., and Rheinberger, M.A. "Mal de Debarquement." *Archives of Otolaryngology-Head and Neck Surgery, 25*(6):615-620, 1999.

Herdman, S.J. *Vestibular Rehabilitation.* Second edition. Philadelphia: F.A. Davis Company, 2000.

Mair, IW. The mal de Debarquement syndrome. *Journal of Audiological Medicine,* 5:21-25, 1996.

Murphy, T.P. "Mal de Debarquement syndrome: a forgotten entity?" *Otolaryngology-Head and Neck Surgery, 109:*10-13, 1993.

Teitelbaum, P. "Mal de Debarquement syndrome: a case report." *Journal of Travel Medicine,* 9(1):51-52, 2002.

Zimbelman J.L., and Walton, T.M. "Vestibular rehabilitation of a patient with persistent Mal de Debarquement." *Physical Therapy Case Reports,* 2(4):129-137, 1999.

Chapter Twenty-eight
Meniere's Disease

Meniere's disease is not the most common vestibular disorder, it isn't even the second most common but it certainly is the name most recognizable to health care professionals. Even if a doctor knows next to nothing about vestibular disorders they know this name. Unfortunately they may also give the name to almost any inner ear disorder that includes vertigo.

Prosper Ménière was the first doctor, in the mid-1800s, to link the symptoms of vertigo, hearing loss and tinnitus to the inner ear rather than the brain. His name has been linked with the three symptoms, attacks of vertigo, hearing loss and ringing in the ears (tinnitus), ever since. (Ear fullness, also called aural fullness, is now considered an important symptom as well).

In an attempt to bring some order and consistency to the diagnosis and reporting of Meniere's Disease treatments the Committee on Hearing and Equilibrium of the American Academy of Otolaryngology-Head and Neck Surgery first published guidelines in 1978. Updates were also published in 1985 and again in 1995.

Currently the Committee defines Meniere's disease as the idiopathic syndrome of endolymphatic hydrops. Broken down:

Idiopathic: No known cause
Syndrome: A group of symptoms
Endolymphatic: Refers to the inner ear fluid endolymph
Hydrops: Swelling

In plane English Meniere's disease is a group of symptoms with no known cause that seems to include having too much endolymph in the inner ear.

Technical point: If the cause is known the disorder can no longer be called Meniere's disease.

The most recent guidelines published in 1995 no longer use the following terms: Meniere's syndrome, vestibular Meniere's disease or cochlear Meniere's disease. Instead they suggest, after all other possible diagnoses have been ruled out, use of the following diagnostic scale:

Possible Meniere's disease: Symptoms include either an episode or episodes of vertigo without hearing loss OR hearing loss and disequilibrium without vertigo.

Probable Meniere's Disease: One episode of vertigo and hearing loss (on testing) and either tinnitus or aural fullness, all in the same ear.
Definite Meniere's disease: Two or more attacks of vertigo lasting 20 or more minutes, hearing loss (on testing) at least once, tinnitus or aural fullness all in the same ear.
Certain Meniere's Disease: Consists of the presence of definite Meniere's disease during life and the finding of endolymphatic hydrops after death.

Meniere's disease can be divided roughly into two phases, early and late. A textbook case of early Meniere's disease would look like this: You suddenly feel a bit off, have enough time to sit or lay down and then vertigo begins. The vertigo may be quite violent and usually occurs along with hearing loss, tinnitus and/or aural fullness, all lasting 20 minutes to 24 hours. After the attack stops you can get up and move about, sometimes without much difficulty but other times having to walk slowly and hold on to things. The hearing loss and tinnitus may linger.

The pattern of attacks varies greatly. They can last from 20 minutes to 24 hours and might appear every day or two, or once or twice a month or years can go by between attacks in some folks. Attacks come and go without apparent rhyme or reason although some people feel their symptoms are linked to stress. Not only does this lack of pattern cause uncertainty in people's lives, it also makes it difficult to figure out if a treatment is working since the attacks stop on their own so frequently.

During late Meniere's the hearing loss and tinnitus are constant and the spontaneous, violent vertigo may be replaced instead by a milder more constant vertigo, unsteadiness and/or feeling of imbalance.

In theory Meniere's disease is a diagnosis of exclusion—testing should be done for all possible causes of the symptoms before the diagnosis is decided upon. Some doctors feel a glycerol test or the electrocochleogram, ECOG, can help determine if excess endolymph is present but neither is a slam-dunk. Some experts feel an abnormal ECOG just means something's wrong, not what.

In practice many doctors make this diagnosis first if vertigo, hearing loss and tinnitus or aural pressure are present. If the diet change and diuretics don't work then they might think about looking for other possible explanations.

Since Meniere's disease is idiopathic the cause isn't known and can't be treated. Instead most doctors in the U.S. go after the assumed affect of the Meniere's disease, the endolymphatic hydrops. This is done with a low sodium diet (anywhere from 1 to 4 grams daily) and/or water pills (diuretics).

Outside the U.S. Meniere's disease is routinely treated with betahistine (Serc). Another treatment more common outside the U.S. is the insertion of an ear tube so the middle ear pressure can be equal to the pressure outside the ear all the time.

The use of pressure has been studied in Sweden for decades and the Meniett machine is the product of that research. Food and Drug Administration approval has been granted and the Meniett is now also available in the U.S. Before treatments can begin an ear tube is inserted through the eardrum in an office procedure. Then, at home, treatments are done for a few minutes a couple of times a day for a few weeks.

If a medical approach to Meniere's disease doesn't help, no treatable cause can be found, and the symptoms are so severe they interfere with the ability to live normally surgery may be suggested. Surgery is almost never the first treatment offered because it can't cure the disease and about the best that can be hoped for is that the disabling episodes of violent vertigo will end. Surgery also has the additional potential for complications and problems.

The most controversial surgical procedures are the endolymphatic shunt, endolymphatic valve and endolymphatic decompression. All are done in an attempt to reduce the amount of endolymph in the ear.

A treatment gaining in popularity is intratympanic or transtympanic gentamicin injection. This treatment aims to destroy enough of the vestibular areas to stop the vertigo. Some doctors feel it also can stop the progression of hearing loss and tinnitus but the jury is still out on that.

Two surgeries aimed at stopping vestibular signals from reaching the brain are the vestibular nerve section and the labyrinthectomy.

About 2/3 of people with Meniere's disease will be able to continue on with their lives needing only diet changes and/or medication. About 1/3 have enough problems and disability to warrant gentamicin treatments or surgery. Nobody knows for sure how many people will go on to develop Meniere's in the second ear but estimates of 1/3 and higher are often mentioned.

Hearing loss and tinnitus are usually not improved by surgery. Tinnitus can be treated with medical treatments such as masking, tinnitus retraining therapy or drugs. Ear fullness might just go away or improve with or without treatment.

If you have this disorder or think you might, there are several organizations you can get information and moral support from: The Vestibular Disorders Association (VEDA), PO Box 13305, Portland, OR 97213-0305, Phone (24-hour voice mail): (800) 837-8428 and (503) 229-7705, Fax: (503) 229-8064 and E-mail: memberinfo@vestibular.org and The Meniere's Network at the Ear Foundation, PO Box 330867, Nashville, TN 37203, Phone Toll Free (voice/TDD): 1-800-545-HEAR, Phone (voice/TDD): (615) 627-2724, Fax (615) 627-2728, info@earfoundation. org

References and Reading List:
There are a number of Meniere's disease books available:
Haybach, P.J. *Meniere's Disease: what you need to know.* Portland, OR: Vestibular Disorders Association, 1998.

Harris, J.P. *Meniere's Disease.* Hague, The Netherlands: Kugler Publications, 1999.

Otolaryngologic Clinics of North America. "Pathogenesis of Meniere's Disease: Treatment Considerations." 35, 2002.

Other sources:
Abou-Halawa, A.S., and Poe, D.S. "Efficacy of increased gentamicin concentration for intratympanic injection therapy in Meniere's Disease." *Otology and Neurotology,* 23(4):494-503, 2002.

Akagi, H., Yuen, K., Maeda, Y., Fukushima, K., Kariya, S., Orita, Y., Kataoka, Y., Ogawa, T., and Nishizaki, K. "Meniere's disease in childhood." *International Journal of Pediatric Otorhinolaryngology,* 61(3):259-264, 2001.

Anderson, J.P., and Harris, J.P. "Impact of Meniere's disease on quality of life." *Otology and Neurotology,* 22(6):888-94, 2001.

Baloh, R.W. "Prosper Meniere and his disease." *Archives of Neurology,* 58(7):1151-1156, 2001.

Ballester, M., Liard, P., Vibert, D., and Hausler, R. "Meniere's disease in the elderly." *Otology and Neurotology,* 23(1):73-78, 2002.

Beasley, N.J., and Jones, N.S. "Meniere's disease: evolution of a definition." *Journal of Laryngology and Otology,* 110(12):1107-1113, 1996.

Claes, J., and Van de Heyning, P.H. "A review of medical treatment for Meniere's disease." *Auris Nasus Larynx,* 29(2):115-119, 2002.

"Committee on Hearing and Equilibrium guidelines for the diagnosis and evaluation of therapy in Meniere's disease." American Academy of Otolaryngology-Head and Neck Foundation, Inc., *Otolaryngology-Head and Neck Surgery,* 113(3):181-185, 1995.

De Kleine, E., Mateijsen, D.J., Wit, H.P., and Albers, F.W. "Evoked otoacoustic emissions in patients with Meniere's Disease." *Otology and Neurotololgy,* 23(4):510-516, 2002.

Fung, K., Xie, Y., Hall, S.F., Lillicrap, D.P., and Taylor, S.A. "Genetic basis of familial Meniere's disease." *Journal of Otolaryngology,* 31(1):1-4, 2002.

Gacek, R.R., and Gacek, M.R. "Meniere's disease: a form of vestibular ganglionitis." *Advances in Otorhinolaryngology,* 60:67-79, 2002.

Havia, M., Kentala, E., and Pyykko, I. "Hearing loss and tinnitus in Meniere's disease." *Acta Otolaryngologica,* Supplement 544:34-39, 2000.

Hollis, L., and Bottrill, I. "Meniere's disease." *Hospital Medicine,* 60(8):574-577, 1999.

Hooter, L.J. "Living with Meniere's disease." *Seminars in Perioperative Nursing,* 9(4):185-187, 2000.

Kotimaki, J., Sorri, M., and Muhli, A. "Prognosis of hearing impairment in Meniere's disease." *Acta Otolaryngologica,* Supplement 545:14-18, 2001.

Mira, E. "Betahistine in the treatment of vertigo. History and clinical implications of recent pharmacological researches." *Acta Otorhinolaryngologica Italia,* 21(3 Supplement 66):1-7, 2001.

Smith, W.K., Sankar, V., and Pfleiderer, A.G. "A national survey amongst UK otolaryngologists regarding the treatment of Meniere's disease." *Journal of Laryngology and Otology,* 119(2):102-5, 2005.

Thai-Van, H., Bounaix, M.J., and Fraysse, B. "Meniere's disease: pathophysiology and treatment." *Drugs,* 61(8):1089-1102, 2001.

Thorp, M.A., Shehab, Z.P., Bance, M.L., and Rutka, J.A. "Does evidence-based medicine exist in the treatment of Meniere's disease? A critical review of the last decade of publications." *Clinical Otolaryngology,* 25(6):456-460, 2000.

Chapter Twenty-nine
Migraine

For a couple of centuries now a relationship between headaches and vestibular symptoms, including motion sickness, has been known. A new idea gaining more acceptance among inner ear experts is that people with inner ear symptoms such as vertigo, dizziness, hearing loss and tinnitus may actually be experiencing a migraine, sometimes without a headache. Some of the names in use for this situation are vestibular migraine, migraine equivalent, migraine-associated dizziness and migraine associated vertigo.

Some doctors have embraced this idea with a great deal of gusto, making the diagnosis pretty frequently while others hardly ever make it.

Right now there's no scientific proof that a migraine can cause inner ear symptoms. There's no test for it and no physical changes have been found in the ears of people with the diagnosis. This disorder is based more on a theory or educated guess but one that seems reasonable and is accepted by a number of experts in the field.

There's been a lot of confusion with this disorder since there's no official definition or title nor guidelines for its diagnosis and treatment. One doctor might call one situation and set of symptoms a vestibular migraine while another would give it a totally different name.

Migraine in general is defined in the July 2001 issue of the Medical Clinics of North America as "a chronic condition of recurring attacks of transient focal neurologic symptoms, headache, or both. The headache is so intense that it 1) interferes with the physical ability to function, sometimes requiring bed rest, and 2) interferes with the functioning of other systems in the body resulting in many associated symptoms."

A migraine is more than a headache. It's a complex topic with entire books devoted to it. The small bit of information in this chapter just barely skims the surface.

In general, 18% of American woman and 6% of American men experience migraines, usually between age 30 and 45. Of these, 25% have some sort of dizziness or vertigo before, during, after or between migraines.

Why people develop migraines is unknown although they do run in some families so genetics probably have a role in some people. Most of the theories attempting to explain what happens during a migraine include a temporary problem in circulation and an inappropriate release of chemicals. The symptoms of a vestibular migraine are thought to be coming from a circulation or chemical effect on the inner ear, the vestibulocochlear nerve or on the vestibular and/or hearing areas of the brain.

There are four general categories of migraines:

- Migraine with an aura
- Migraine without an aura
- Ophthalmologic migraine
- Retinal migraine

The migraines associated most commonly with vestibular symptoms are migraines with an aura, migraines without an aura and a sub-category of migraines with an aura called basilar migraines. An aura is a symptom or collection of symptoms occurring before the migraine begins in earnest. The most common symptom is visual and can be the illusion of looking through a tunnel, holes in the visual field, flashing lights and that sort of thing.

Rather than occurring totally out of the blue migraines can be brought on by a particular event or experience called a trigger. Known triggers include sleep deprivation, altered sleep pattern, motion sickness, oversleep, barometric changes, menstruation, birth control pills, hormone replacement therapy, beer, red wine, champagne, caffeine, cured meats, monosodium glutamate, NutraSweet, strong cheeses, yogurt, pickled foods, cigar smoke, perfume, candle shops, glare, bright lights, striped or geometric shapes, fasting, exercise, stress, chocolate, ice cream, tyramine, nitrates, upper respiratory infection, cigarette smoke, odors, trauma, x-ray dyes and certain drugs.

Migraine is a disorder defined by a list of symptoms rather than by tests or the presence of recognizable and measurable physical changes. The diagnosis is based upon the history and signs/symptoms. A doctor's belief system also comes into play here. If they don't buy into the theory of a "vestibular" migraine they won't make the diagnosis.

The inner ear type symptoms thought to occur in this disorder are violent spinning vertigo, vomiting, dry heaving, extreme motion intolerance, constant unsteadiness or imbalance, unbalanced feeling, and/or motion related symptoms. Hearing loss and tinnitus are also possible but thought to be uncommon. When they do occur it's in both ears about 2/3 of the time. The migraine can last minutes to hours with some vestibular symptoms going on for days. If the migraines come frequently a person may never be symptom free.

A person may have headaches and dizziness at the same time, headaches and dizziness at different times, a family history of migraine, no headaches at all, or a personal history of migraines that are no longer occurring.

Vestibular migraine is treated like other migraines. Drugs can be used to stop an attack once it's in progress or to prevent them from occurring. Ergots (ergotamine), triptans (Almotriptan, eletriptan, etc.), anti-inflammatories (aspirin, naproxen), calcium-entry blockers (verapamil, flunarizine), tricyclic antidepressants (amitriptyline, pizotifen), anti-convulsants and methysergide are all in use.

Vestibular rehabilitation therapy has been found to be helpful in some people. Unfortunately if hearing loss occurs there is no treatment to restore it.

Another migraine, basilar migraines, (also called basilar artery migraines) can also cause vertigo. The problem with these is thought to occur in the basilar artery that supplies the brain and inner ear with their blood. It most commonly occurs in females in their teen years.

At least two of the following symptoms must be present for the diagnosis of basilar migraine to be made: visual symptoms in both eyes, trouble swallowing, vertigo, hearing loss, double vision, or uncoordinated walking.

References and Reading List:

Baloh, R.W., Jacobson, K.J., and Fife, T. "Familial vestibulopathy: a new dominantly inherited syndrome." *Neurology*, 40:20-25, 1994.

Baloh, R.W., Foster, C.A., Yue, Q., and Nelson, S.F. "Familial migraine with vertigo and essential tremor." *Neurology,* 146(2):458-460, 1996.

Bikhazi, P., Jackson, C., and Ruckenstein, M.J. "Efficacy of antimigrainous therapy in the treatment of migraine-associated dizziness." *American Journal of Otology,* 18:350-354, 1997.

Cass, S.P., Furman, J.M., and Ankerstjerne, J.K. "Migraine-related vestibulopathy." *Annals of Otology, Rhinology, and Laryngology,* 106:182-189, 1997.

Cutrer, F.M., and Baloh, RW. "Migraine associated dizziness." *Headache,* 32:300-304, 1992.

Johnson, G.D. "Medical management of migraine-related dizziness and vertigo." *Laryngoscope,* 108 (Supplement 85):1-28, 1998.

Kayan, A., and Hood, J.D. "Neuro-otological manifestations of migraine." *Brain,* 107:1123, 1984.

Kuritzky, A., Toglias, U.J., and Thomas, D. "Vestibular function in Migraine." *Headache,* 21:110-112, 1981.

Kuritsky, A., Ziegler, D., and Hassanein, R. "Vertigo, motion sickness and migraine." *Headache,* 21:227-231, 1981.

Lee, H., Lopez, I., Ishiyama, A., and Baloh, R.W. "Can migraine damage the inner ear?" *Archives of Neurology,* 57(11):1631-1634, 2000.

Neuhauser, H., Leopold, M., von Brevern, M., Arnold, G., and Lempert, T. "The interrelations of migraine, vertigo, and migrainous vertigo." *Neurology,* 27:56(4):436-441, 2001.

Olsson, J.E. "Neurotologic findings in basilar migraine." *Laryngoscope,* 101:1-41, 1991.

Radtke, A., Lempert, T., Gresty, M.A., Brookes, G.B., Bronstein, A.M., and Neuhauser, H. "Migraine and Meniere's disease: is there a link?" *Neurology,* 59:1700-1704, 2002.

Rassekh, C.H., and Harker, L.A. "The prevalence of migraine in Meniere's disease." *Laryngoscope,* 102:135-138, 1992.

Slater, R. "Benign recurrent vertigo." *Journal of Neurology, Neurosurgery and Psychiatry,* 42:363, 1979.

Spierings, E.L. "Mechanism of migraine and actions of antimigraine." *Medical Clinics of North America,* 85(4):943-958, 2001.

Stahl, J.S., and Daroff, R.B. "Time for more attention to migrainous vertigo?" *Neurology,* 27:56(4):428-429, 2001.

Thakar, A., Anjaneyulu, C., and Deka, R.C. "Vertigo syndromes and mechanisms in migraine." *Journal of Laryngology and Otology,* 115(10):782-787, 2001.

Tusa, R.J. "Diagnosis and management of neuro-otologic disorders due to migraine." *ICS Medical Report,* July 1999.

Virre, E.S., and Baloh, R.W. "Migraine as a cause of sudden hearing loss." *Headache,* 36(1):24-28, 1996.

Whitney, S.L., Wrisley, D.M., Brown, K.E., and Furman, J.M. "Physical therapy for migraine-related vestibulopathy and vestibular dysfunction with history of migraine." *Laryngoscope,* 110(9):1528-1534, 2000.

Chapter Thirty
Multiple Sclerosis

Multiple sclerosis does not affect the inner ear but can damage the vestibulocochlear nerve in the area where it enters the brain. Hearing loss occurs in around 10% of all people with MS and vertigo occurs at some point in time in as many as 50%. Of all the people diagnosed with MS, vertigo will be the very first symptom felt by 5%.

Technical point: The vestibulocochlear nerve runs from the inner ear to the brain supplying hearing and balance information.

There is no specific treatment for damage to the vestibulocochlear nerve other than the standard treatments for the various types of MS.

There isn't a single test that can both diagnose MS and determine accurately if it has damaged the vestibulocochlear nerve. Instead the usual tests for diagnosing MS are done, including MRI, in addition to vestibular testing.

References and Reading List:

Alpini, D., Caputo, D., Pugnetti. L., Giuliano, D.A., and Cesarani, A. "Vertigo and multiple sclerosis: aspects of differential diagnosis." *Neurological Science,* Supplement 22, 2:S84-87, 2001.

Daugherty, W.T., Lederman, R.J., Nodar, R.H., and Conomy J.P. "Hearing loss in multiple sclerosis." *Archives of Neurology,* 40(1):33-35, 1983.

Downey, D.L., Stahl, J.S., Bhidayasiri, R., Derwenskus, J., Adams, N.L., Ruff, R.L., and Leigh, R.J. "Saccadic and vestibular abnormalities in multiple sclerosis: sensitive clinical signs of brainstem and cerebellar involvement." *Annals of the New York Academy of Science,* 956:438-440, 2002.

Frohman, E.M., Zhang, H., Dewey, R.B., Hawker, K.S., Racke, M.K., and Frohman, T.C. "Vertigo in MS: utility of positional and particle repositioning maneuvers." *Neurology,* 28:55(10):1566-1569, 2000.

Gass, A., Steinke, W., Schwartz, A., and Hennerici, M.G. "High resolution magnetic resonance imaging in peripheral vestibular dysfunction in multiple sclerosis." *Journal of Neurology, Neurosurgery, and Psychiatry,* 65(6):945, 1998.

Gstoettner, W., Swoboda, H., Muller, C., and Burian, M. "Preclinical detection of initial vestibulocochlear abnormalities in a patient with multiple sclerosis." *European Archives of Otorhinolaryngology, 250(1):40-43, 1993.*

Herrera, W.G. "Vestibular and other balance disorders in multiple sclerosis. Differential diagnosis of disequilibrium and topognostic localization." *Neurologic Clinics,* 8(2):407-420, 1990.

Molteni, R.A. "Vertigo as a presenting symptom of multiple sclerosis in childhood.*" American Journal of Disabled Children,* 131(5):553-554, 1977.

Ozunlu, A., Mus, N., and Gulhan, M. "Multiple sclerosis: a cause of sudden hearing loss." *Audiology,* 37(1):52-58, 1998.

Sasaki, O., Ootsuka, K., Taguchi, K., and Kikukawa, M. "Multiple sclerosis presented acute hearing loss and vertigo." *Journal of Otorhinolaryngology and It's Related Specialties,* 56(1):55-59, 1994.

Schick, B., Brors, D., Koch, O., Schafers, M., and Kahle, G., "Magnetic resonance imaging in patients with sudden hearing loss, tinnitus and vertigo."*Otology and Neurotology,* 22(6):808-12, 2001.

Weissman, J.L., and Hirsch, B.E. "Magnetic resonance imaging in patients with sudden hearing loss, tinnitus and vertigo." *Otology and Neurotology,* 22(6):808-812, 2001.

Williams, N.P., Roland, P.S., and Yellin, W. "Vestibular evaluation in patients with early multiple sclerosis." *American Journal of Otology,* 18(1):93-100, 1997.

Chapter Thirty-one
Otosclerosis

Otosclerosis is a bone disorder affecting the normal growth cycle of the stapes, the little middle ear bone that connects to the oval window, a membrane covered opening between the inner and middle ears.

Bone is a living tissue that renews itself. New bone is constantly made and old bone taken away by special cells. Something goes wrong with this process in otosclerosis.

The cause of otosclerosis isn't known. Some research points to an inflammatory disease such as an autoimmune reaction or a virus such as the one causing measles. It's also known to run in some families and research has discovered three different problem areas on chromosomes responsible for otosclerosis. If a parent has the disorder the chance of their child developing it is 50%.

Hearing loss, often in both ears, is the problem most commonly bringing the disorder to a person's attention. There are two forms of otosclerosis, stapedial and cochlear. Stapedial otosclerosis damages the stapes bone causing a conductive hearing loss. In the less common cochlear form the hearing loss is sensorineural (also called nerve deafness). The two are often found together creating both types of hearing loss in the same person. In addition to hearing loss, tinnitus is also common.

It's been suggested that a vestibular form exists as well but proof of this isn't as good as the evidence for the stapedial and cochlear forms of the disease.

A large percentage of people with otosclerosis have vestibular symptoms. Episodes typically consist of a rocking sensation lasting for 60 seconds or less that may be brought on or worsened by head movement. Unsteadiness while walking and in the dark can also be experienced.

The exact reason vestibular symptoms occur isn't known. The stapes may damage the membrane-covered opening into the inner ear or maybe even create a perilymphatic fistula in which inner ear fluid leaks into the middle ear. It also seems reasonable to figure if the disease can affect the cochlea and disturb hearing it can do the same thing in the vestibular areas.

Otosclerosis is diagnosed with the history and examination, standard hearing tests and imaging tests like the CT and MRI. In addition approximately 10% of people with otosclerosis also have a visible change that can be seen by looking at the eardrum with an otoscope.

Treatments include medical and surgical approaches. Sodium fluoride is sometimes prescribed, many times along with vitamin D and calcium. At least one doctor has suggested, in a medical journal, the use of etidronate (Didronel) instead. Hearing aids can help with hearing in the stapedial form of the disease.

In the U.S. stapedectomy surgery can be done to restore hearing or stop the progression of hearing loss when the otosclerosis is damaging the stapes. The stapes bone is removed and replaced with an artificial one. Unfortunately the surgery itself causes deafness in 1% of the people who undergo it and can actually cause vestibular symptoms.

Like all surgery in the middle ear these surgeries can cause deafness or hearing loss, vestibular symptoms, changes in the ability to taste food and drink, tinnitus and facial nerve damage. There are also the usual risks of surgery and anesthesia including infection.

A textbook case of otosclerosis would include hearing loss in both ears in a twenty or thirty year old with a family history of the disorder. This person would be slightly more likely to be a woman than a man and would have a slightly greater than 50% chance of having vestibular symptoms. Ten percent of all Caucasians have otosclerosis but only 1% seek treatment due to hearing loss. The numbers of non-whites are much lower.

For help understanding and living with a hearing loss check out Self-help for the Hard of Hearing on the Internet at www.shhh.org or write them at: 7910 Woodmont Ave, Suite 1200, Bethesda, Maryland 20814, 301-657-2248 Voice, 301-657-2249 TTY and 301-913-9413 Fax

References and Reading List:

Birch, L., and Elbrond, O. "Stapedectomy and vertigo." *Clinical Otolaryngology,* 10(4):217-223, 1985.

Brookler, K.H., and Tanyeri, H. "Edidronate for the neurotologic symptoms of otosclerosis: preliminary study." *Ear Nose Throat Journal,* 76(6):372-378, 1997.

Chen, W., Campbell, C.A., Green, G.E., Van Den Bogaert, K., Komodikis, C., Manolidis, L.S., Aconomou, E., Kyamides, Y., Christodoulou, K., Faghel, C., Giguere C.M., Alford, R.L., Manolidis, S., Van Camp, G., and Smith, R.J. "Linkage of otosclerosis to a third locus (OTSC3) on human chromosome 6p21.3-22.3" *Journal of Medical Genetics,* 39(7):473-477, 2002.

Chole, R.A., and McKenna, M. "Pathophysiology of otosclerosis." *Otology and Neurotology,* 22(2):249-257, 2001.

Goh, J.P., Chan, L.L., and Tan, T.Y. "MRI of cochlear otosclerosis. *British Journal of Radiology,* 75(894):502-505, 2002.

Li, W., Schachern, P.A., and Paparella, M.M. "Extensive otosclerosis and endolymphatic hydrops: histopathologic study of temporal bones." *American Journal of Otolaryngology,* 15(2):158-161, 1994.

Lolov, S.R., Encheva, V.I., Kyurkchiev, S.D., Edrev, G.E., and Kehayov, I.R. "Antimeasles immunoglobulin G in sera of patients with otosclerosis is lower than that in healthy people." *Otology and Neurotology,* 22(6):766-770, 2001.

Niedermeyer, H.P., Arnold, W., Schuster, M., Baumann, C., Kramer, J., Neubert, W.J., and Sedlmeier, R. "Persistent measles virus infection and otosclerosis," *Annals of Otology, Rhinology, and Laryngology,* 110(10):897-903, 2001.

Niedermeyer, H.P., and Arnold, W. "Etiopathogenesis of otosclerosis." *Journal of Otorhinolaryngology and It's Related Specialties,* 64(2):114-119, 2002.

Raut, V.V., Toner, J.G., Kerr, A.G., and Stevenson, M. "Management of otosclerosis in the UK." *Clinical Otolaryngology,* 27(2):113-119, 2002.

Shea, J.J. Jr., Ge, X., and Orchik, D.J. "Endolymphatic hydrops associated with otosclerosis." *American Journal of Otology,* 15(3):348-357, 1994.

Yoon, T.H., Paparella, M.M., and Schachern, P.A. "Otosclerosis involving the vestibular aqueduct and Meniere's disease." *Otolaryngology-Head and Neck Surgery,* 103(1):107-112, 1990.

Chapter Thirty-two
Ototoxicity

Ototoxicity literally means ear poisoning but in practice health care professionals only use the term to refer to poisoning of the inner ear(s). The poisoning can affect hearing, balance or both. Unfortunately some health care pros view it as a disorder of hearing alone.

This chapter will cover unintentional or accidental ototoxicity. Information about the intentional use of ototoxic drugs to kill inner ear hair cells can be found later in the book.

This is not the most common inner ear disorder but it is one of the best understood. It isn't a theory or idea, it's a fact backed up with research. This poisoning occurs in animals as well as humans, making it easier than most disorders to study.

Ototoxicity can affect the cochlea, the vestibular areas of the inner ear or both. Ototoxicity occurring in the cochlea is sometimes referred to as cochleotoxicity and in the vestibular areas as vestibulotoxicity.

It can be a temporary problem or permanent. When temporary, ototoxicity is an annoyance, when permanent it is life altering and possibly disabling. Whether or not it's permanent depends upon the drug, how it was placed into the body and the health and genetics of the person receiving the drug. Some drugs are virtually always temporary and others permanent. They can affect hearing, balance or both.

The Most Common Ototoxic Drug Groups Are:

- Aspirin and quinine, and the drugs containing them
  These have been known to cause temporary tinnitus (or increase tinnitus in someone who already has it) and/or mild hearing loss since the late 1800's. This affect generally passes once the drug is stopped.
- Cisplatin
  Cisplatin, an anticancer drug, usually causes permanent hearing loss that's massive at times.
- Loop Diuretics
  The loop diuretics, a specific family of anti-water drugs, can also cause temporary tinnitus and hearing loss. These stop once the drug dosage is reduced or stopped. These are the strongest diuretic or water pills available and include Lasix (furosemide), Bumex, Demadex and ethacrynic acid.
  When loop diuretics are given along with another ototoxic drug class, the

aminoglycoside antibiotics (See below), it's thought to increase the chance of an irreversible problem developing.
- Aminoglycosides
An entire family of antibiotics, the aminoglycosides, can cause permanent vestibular and/or hearing damage. These antibiotics are usually given IV for serious infections but can also be given by other methods such as ear or eye drops, pill form, in breathing sprays, or as an ointment.

The generic names of the aminoglycosides are gentamicin, streptomycin, tobramycin, neomycin, amikacin, netilmicin, kanamycin, paromomycin, dibekacin, framycetin, ribostamycin, and sisomicin.

By far, the drug causing the most cases of permanent vestibular ototoxicity is gentamicin, when given intravenously. It's used extensively in the U.S. to prevent or treat serious infections and used in China, India and some other locations for less serious infections.

When given as eye drops, or as an ointment on a small bit of skin, ototoxicity doesn't occur, but if dropped into an ear that has an ear tube or a ripped eardrum it can. Breathing sprays may also cause ototoxicity because the drug can enter the blood stream through the lungs. Pills given by mouth for months or years on end can also cause toxicity.

Vestibular ototoxicity is a loss or reduction in function. Balance signals aren't sent differently nor do they come and go like in disorders such as Meniere's disease. Instead, they are less in number or gone. The loss is usually the same in both ears, a fact that's useful in making the diagnosis.

The symptoms someone experiences with vestibular ototoxicity depend upon the speed with which the loss occurs, the amount of loss and if the loss is two-sided or one-sided. Rapid damage and one-sided damage generally begin with the most dramatic symptoms. Symptoms from a one sided loss are usually only a short-term problem. (Weeks to months)

If the loss is one-sided, massive and sudden, there's violent vertigo for a few days with nausea, vomiting and nystagmus. The really strong, sickening symptoms last for 2 to 3 days and then slowly simmer down.

A person should be walking with help around day 4 or 5 and independent in a week or so, if they don't have another condition stopping the natural progression of what vestibular scientists call vestibular compensation. The nystagmus will also calm down over a week or two and then disappear as well.

At the end of the compensation process a person will get totally back to normal, as long as the brain is normal and the opposite ear is working properly.

The typical case of vestibular ototoxicity is one where both ears are affected at the same time. As goofy as it may sound, the first symptoms of two-eared toxicity may not be as dramatic as the one-sided variety.

Once the poisoning is in full swing balance will be difficult while walking or standing in daylight and impossible in darkness. Walking may look more like staggering, the legs may be placed more widely apart and a person may have to hold onto walls, furniture, etc. to move around. If severe enough, walking may only be possible with someone holding them up or when using a walker.

Vision will bounce during head movement and sometimes in synch with heartbeat. This bouncing vision is called oscillopsia and occurs because the vestibulocular reflex (VOR) can't work when the brain isn't getting enough vestibular signals. Oscillopsia may make it seem like the eyes are bouncing around like crazy. Quite the opposite is actually the case; the eyes aren't being automatically positioned during head movement.

At the end of two or three years of relearning balance the disturbed vision becomes the most disabling problem a person with virtually no vestibular balance system has.

Although ototoxicity is a proven fact no slam-dunk test exists for diagnosing ototoxicity in a specific person. If testing shows reduced or lost function in both ears and there's a history of ototoxic drug use the diagnosis may be made. A doctor may order up an ENG, rotational testing and/or VEMP to document the reduced function.

There is no cure for ototoxicity. The only way to prevent it is not using ototoxic drugs in the first place, something that isn't always possible. Once the ototoxicity has occurred the only treatment is to stop the offending drug, when possible, and begin vestibular rehabilitation

This treatment helps in two ways: it gets the most use out of the remaining vestibular function and helps in the process of learning how to balance oneself using mainly vision and proprioception. It takes from 18 months to a couple of years after the start of serious rehabilitation before the level of permanent disability can be determined or predicted.

Some Frequently Asked Questions:
What are the names of all the potentially ototoxic drugs?
The drugs already discussed in this chapter are undoubtedly ototoxic. Many other drugs appear on ototoxic drug lists but are usually there due to casual observation, not scientific proof.

How many people develop permanent, disabling ototoxicity?
Isn't that the $64,000 question? Unfortunately, to almost all health care professionals, ototoxicity conjures up visions of hearing loss, not a balance disorder. Testing for vestibular damage during ototoxic drug treatment is seldom done so nobody knows how large the problem of vestibular ototoxicity is.

Why are aminoglycoside antibiotics still on the market?
Good question with at least three answers. These drugs save lives when given for serious infections, they are cheap to use and most doctors find ototoxicity to be an acceptable risk. Unfortunately most of them have no idea what the risk really includes.

If you have gentamicin ototoxicity or think you might, there is one organization trying to provide moral support: Wobblers Anonymous, www.wobblers.com.

References and Reading List:
Arslan, E., Orzan, E., and Santarelli, R. "Global problem of drug-induced hearing loss." *Annals of the New York Academy of Science*, 28:884:1-14, 1999.

Bates, D.E., Beaumont, S.J., and Baylis, B.W. "Ototoxity induced by gentamicin and furosemide." *Annals of Pharmacotherapy*, 36(3):446-451, 2002.

Bath, A.P., Walsh, R.M., Bance, M.L., and Rutka, J.A. "Ototoxicity of topical gentamicin preparations." *Laryngoscope*, 109(7 Pt 1):1088-1093, 1999.

Becvarovski, Z., Michaelides, E.M., Kartush, J.M., Bojrab, D.I., and LaRouere, M.J. "Rapid elevation of gentamicin levels in the human labyrinth following intravenous administration." *Laryngoscope*, 112(7):1163-1165, 2002.

Black, F.O., Gianna-Poulin, C., and Pesznecker, S.C. "Recovery from vestibular ototoxicity." *Otology and Neurotology*, 22(5):662-671, 2001.

Fischel-Ghodsian, N. "Genetic factors in aminoglycoside toxicity." *Annals of the New York Academy of Sciences,* 28;884:99-109, 1999.

Freeman, S., Priner, R., Elidan, J., and Sohmer, H. "Objective method for differentiating between drug-induced vestibulotoxicity and cochleotoxicity." *Otology and Neurotology,* 22(1):70-75, 2001.

Hinojosa, R., Nelson, E.G., Lerner, S.A., Redleaf, M.I., and Schramm, D.R. "Aminoglycoside ototoxicity: a human temporal bone study." *Laryngoscope,* 111(10):1797-1805, 2001.

Kaplan, D.M., Hehar, S.S., Bance, M.L., and Rutka, J.A. "Intentional ablation of vestibular function using commercially available topical gentamicin-betamethasone eardrops in patients with Meniere's disease: further evidence for topical eardrop ototoxicity." *Laryngoscope,* 112(4):689-695, 2002.

Miman, M.C., Ozturan, O., Iraz, M., Erdem, T., and Olmez, E. "Amikacin ototoxicity enhanced by Ginkgo biloba extract (EGb 761)." *Hearing Research,* 169(1-2):121-129, 2002.

Nakashima, T., Teranishi, M., Hibi, T., Kobayashi, M., and Umemura, M. "Vestibular and cochlear toxicity of aminoglycosides—a review." *Acta Otolaryngologica,* 120(8):904-911, 2000.

Palomar, G.V., Abdulghani, M.F., Bodetm A.E., Andreu, M.L., and Palomar, A.V. "Drug-induced otoxicity: current status." *Acta Otolaryngologica,* 121(5):569-572, 2001.

Palomar, G.V., and Palomar, A.V. "Are some ear drops ototoxic or potentially ototoxic?" *Acta Otolaryngologica,* 121(5):565-568, 2001.

Seidman, M.D., and Jacobson, G.P. "Update on tinnitus." *Otolaryngologic Clinics of North America,* 29(3):455-465, 1996.

Smith, P.F. "Are vestibular hair cells excited to death by aminoglycoside antibiotics?" *Journal of Vestibular Research,* 10(1):1-5, 2000.

Smith, P.F. "Pharmacology of the vestibular system." *Current Opinions in Neurology, 13(1):31-37, 2000.*

Stavroulaki, P., Vossinakis, I.C., Dinopoulou, D., Doudounakis, S., Adamopoulos, G., and Apostolopoulos, N. "Otoacoustic emissions for monitoring aminoglycoside-induced ototoxicity in children with cystic fibrosis." *Archives of Otolaryngology-Head and Neck Surgery,* 128(2):150-155, 2002.

Tange, R.A. "Ototoxicity." *Adverse Drug Reactions and Toxicological Review,* 17(2-3):75-89, 1998.

Wu, W.J., Sha, S.H., and Schacht, J. "Recent advances in understanding aminoglycoside ototoxicity and its prevention." *Audiology and Neurootology,* 7(3):171-174, 2002.

Chapter Thirty-three
Perilymphatic Fistula

A perilymphatic fistula (PLF) is an abnormal opening in the inner ear that leaks perilymph, one of the two inner ear fluids. This opening can be between the inner ear and the middle ear or between the perilymph and endolymph fluid compartments within the inner ear. Other names for this condition include perilymph fistula and PLF.

People can be born with ear bone malformations such as Mondini malformation that lead to PLF's or they can occur for other reasons like the growth of a cholesteatoma. Virtually all experts will agree that the extremes in pressure possible during scuba diving and flying in an unpressurized cabin can create one of these abnormal openings, many believe it can occur from head trauma, some feel it can be caused by sneezing, coughing, sniffing and straining on the toilet and a few feel it can occur spontaneously, out of the blue.

There really isn't a textbook profile of symptoms associated with it. Many are possible and can occur in any and every pattern imaginable. They can come in episodes or be fairly constant. Symptoms can include feelings of imbalance, nausea, fatigue, vertigo, rocking boat feeling, hearing loss, tinnitus, ear fullness, unsteadiness, trouble with memory and thought, headache and sometimes difficulty sleeping.

What usually sets this problem apart from other vestibular disorders is that a number of specific things can bring on or worsen symptoms. These include exercise, straining, lifting, bending over, holding heavy objects, coughing, vomiting, sneezing, swallowing and pressure changes in the external ear canal from flying and weather changes. Loud sounds may also bring on or worsen symptoms.

No easy slam-dunk test exists for this disorder. When a "fistula" test is positive the best that can be said is that pressure changes caused symptoms or abnormal eye movements, not that a PLF did it.

One "fistula" test measures eye movements while air pressure is changed in the canal. In another test balance is checked while the ear canal pressure is changed.

If the tests are negative it doesn't automatically mean there's no fistula, it can mean that the pressure change isn't affecting it right then. If they're positive it doesn't automatically mean there's a fistula either.

Endoscopy, insertion of a small camera into the middle ear through the eardrum, can also be done to look for leaking perilymph (only in the middle ear type of fistula). If a leak is seen the diagnosis can be confirmed and another surgical procedure can be done to place a patch over the opening. Unfortunately if a leak isn't seen PLF can't be ruled out entirely. Endoscopy isn't in widespread use in part because it's expensive, has some risk involved and can be inconclusive.

Treatment isn't a sure thing and depends upon the location, symptoms, and what a doctor believes about PLF's.

When the fistula is totally within the inner ear bed rest with the head higher than the heart can be attempted to help it heal. If that doesn't work there are three approaches: grin and bare it, vestibular suppressant drugs, and surgery to stop all the vestibular signals, good and bad, from leaving the inner ear and traveling to the brain. Unfortunately there is no surgery to repair it.

A fistula between the inner and middle ears can also be treated with bed rest in an attempt to help it heal. Surgery to patch the hole is also available and includes all the usual risks of being put to sleep and having surgery. If hearing loss is occurring and getting worse and worse immediate surgery may be the first option offered in an attempt to prevent the hearing loss from worsening further. This type of surgery doesn't have a good track record in restoring hearing but can be useful in stopping it from getting any worse.

The prognosis for a perilymphatic fistula varies so much no generalization can be made other than this: in many people it's a temporary vestibular nuisance and in others it can be disabling.

References and Reading List:

Black, F.O., Pesznecker, S.C., Norton, T., Fowler, L., Lilly, D.J., Shupert, C., Hemenway, W.G., Peterka, R.J., and Jacobson, E.S. "Surgical management of perilymphatic fistulas: a Portland experience." *American Journal of Otology,* 13(3):254-262, 1992.

Collet, C., Vernet-Maury, E., Miniconi, P., Chanel, J., and Dittmar, A. "Autonomic nervous system activity associated with postural disturbances in patients with perilymphatic fistula: sympathetic or vagal origin?" *Brain Research Bulletin,* 1:53(1):33-43, 2000.

DeJong, A.L. "Congenital perilymphatic fistula." *Archives of Otolaryngology-Head and Neck Surgery,* 124(11):1279-1281, 1998.

Ferber-Viart, C., Postec, F., Duclaux, R., and Dubreuil, C. "Perilymphatic fistula following airbag trauma." *Laryngoscope,* 108(8 Pt 1):1255-1257, 1998.

Fitzgerald, D.C. "Perilymphatic fistula and Meniere's disease. Clinical series and literature review." *Annals of Otology, Rhinology and Laryngology,* 110(5 Pt 1):430-436, 2001.

Fitzgerald, D.C., Getson, P., and Brasseux, C.O. "Perilymphatic fistula: a Washington, DC experience." *Annals of Otology, Rhinology, and Laryngology,* 106(10 Pt 1):830-837, 1997.

Glasscock, M.E., Hart, M.J., Rosdeutscher, J.D., and Bhansali, S.A. "Traumatic perilymphatic fistula: how long can symptoms persist? A follow-up report." *American Journal of Otology,* 13(4):333-338, 1992.

Grimm, R.J., Hemenway, W.G., Lebray, P.R., and Black, F.O. "The perilymph fistula syndrome defined in mild head trauma." *Acta Otolaryngologica,* Supplement 464:1-40, 1989.

Jones, R. "Current status of perilymphatic fistula." *Archives of Otolaryngology-Head and Neck Surgery,* 124(11):1281-1282, 1998.

Kim, S.H., Kazahaya, K., and Handler, S.D. "Traumatic perilymphatic fistulas in children: etiology, diagnosis and management." *International Journal of Pediatric Otorhinolaryngology*, 20:60(2):147-153, 2001.

Kohut, R.I. "Perilymphatic fistulae: more than a century of notions, conjectures, and critical studies." *American Journal of Otology*, 13(1):38-40, 1992.

Kohut, R.I., Hinojosa, R., and Ryu, J.H. "Update on idiopathic perilymphatic fistulas." *Otolaryngologic Clinics of North America*, 29(2):343-352, 1996.

Kohut, R.I., Hinojosa, R., Thompson, J.N., and Ryu, J.H. "Idiopathic perilymphatic fistulae: a temporal bone histopathological study. Clinical, surgical and histopathological correlations." *Acta Otolaryngologica*, Supplement 520 Pt 1:225-234, 1995.

Lehrer, J.F., and Quraishi, A. "Traumatic and perilymphatic fistula PLF." *Journal of Trauma*, 42(2):346-347, 1997.

Maitland, C.G. "Perilymphatic fistula." *Current Neurology and Neuroscience Reports*, 1(5):486-491, 2001.

Meyerhoff, W.L. "Spontaneous perilymphatic fistula: myth or fact." *American Journal of Otology*, 14(5):478-481, 1993.

Naiberg, J.B., Flemming, E., Patterson, M., and Hawke, M. "The perilymphatic fistula: the end of an enigma?" *Journal of Otolaryngology*, 19(4):260-263, 1990.

Pullen, F.W. "Perilymphatic fistula induced by barotrauma." *American Journal of Otology*, 13(3):270-272, 1992.

Sheridan, M.F., Hetherington, H.H., and Hull, J.J. "Inner ear barotrauma from scuba diving." *Ear, Nose, Throat Journal*, 78(3):181, 184, 186-7, 1999.

Weider, D.J. "Treatment and management of perilymphatic fistula: a New Hampshire experience." *American Journal of Otology*, 13(2):158-166, 1992.

Chapter Thirty-four
Shingles

Shingles can occur in any body area including the ear. It's caused by the re-emergence of the chicken pox virus that lingers in all of us once we've had chicken pox. The herpes zoster virus hides along nerves and can spring into action anytime during our lives.

Note: The chicken pox virus is known as varicella zoster and the shingles virus as herpes zoster.

You can only develop shingles if you've had chicken pox in the past, shingles can't be caught from another person. However, adults who have not had chicken pox can develop chicken pox after being exposed to someone with shingles.

When herpes zoster affects the ear it's called herpes zoster oticus. This virus is thought to actually attack a part of the facial nerve (specifically the geniculate ganglion) and then go on to affect the nearby vestibulocochlear nerve. When the herpes zoster virus affects both the facial nerve and vestibulocochlear nerve it may also be referred to as Ramsay-Hunt Syndrome, Ramsay-Hunt Syndrome type I, geniculate neuralgia or nervus intermedius.

The signs and symptoms can be any combination of facial nerve and vestibulocochlear nerve problems and usually involves pain, rash and/or loss of function on one side of the face. Facial weakness or paralysis; blister-like red rash on the ear, in the ear canal, on the face, neck, scalp or in the mouth; burning ear pain, pain under the rash that is strongest when scratching it, numbness and tingling of the external ear, dry mouth, hearing loss, vertigo, nystagmus and tinnitus can also occur in almost any combination.

The strength of the vertigo and length of time it's present depends upon the amount of nerve damage and if it's permanent. In a worse case scenario the flow of vestibular information from the ear stops and doesn't come back. When that flow of vestibular information is suddenly cut off strong vertigo and nystagmus begin along with nausea and vomiting. The first two or three days can be a blur of vertigo and vomiting for many people. Drugs to suppress the vertigo and stop the vomiting are usually needed during that time.

Over the first days to weeks the brain readjusts and changes the way it works so movement and gravity information from only one ear can be used successfully for balance and vestibular reflexes. This begins to occur spontaneously in most people as they look around and move their heads. Vestibular rehabilitation therapy can speed up or help complete this process.

Before the brain changes it's way of using the vestibular information, formally called vestibular compensation, there will be a general feeling of unsteadiness, lightheadedness, spatial disorientation and difficulty with balance in the dark or with the eyes closed. Most people will progress to the point of both feeling and functioning in a normal way with no symptoms.

It's generally diagnosed by the symptoms and the presence of the blister-like rash. The blister fluid can be tested for the presence of the virus and a blood test for antibodies to the virus is also available.

Just like chicken pox, shingles will go away with or without treatment. Unfortunately the damage caused by the virus may be permanent. Antivirus drugs like acyclovir and Famiclovir should be given immediately to combat the virus itself and limit both damage and symptoms. Pain medications and warm, moist compresses can help limit symptoms.

Early treatment with anti-viral drugs and steroids seem to lead to the best end result. If the infection is severe and/or treatment delayed the facial paralysis, deafness and vestibular loss can be permanent.

References and Reading List:

De, S., and Pfleiderer, A.G. "An extreme and unusual variant of Ramsay Hunt syndrome." *Journal of Laryngology and Otology*, 113(7):670-671, 1999.

Furuta, Y., Takasu, T., Suzuki, S., Fukuda, S., Inuyama, Y., and Nagashima, K. "Detection of latent varicella-zoster virus infection in human vestibular and spiral ganglia." *Journal of Medical Virology*, 51(3):214-216, 1997.

Kimitsuki, T., and Komiyama, S. "Ramsay-Hunt syndrome in a 4-year-old child." *European Archives of Otorhinolaryngology*, Supplement 256, 1:S6-7, 1999.

Kinishi, M., Amatsu, M., Mohri, M., Saito, M., Hasegawa, T., and Hasegawa, S. "Acyclovir improves recovery rate of facial nerve palsy in Ramsay Hunt syndrome." *Auris Nasus Larynx*, 28(3):223-226, 2001.

Ko, J.Y., Sheen, T.S., and Hsu, M.M. "Herpes zoster oticus treated with acyclovir and prednisolone: clinical manifestations and analysis of prognostic factors." *Clinical Otolaryngology*, 25(2):139-142, 2000.

Kuhweide, R., Van de Steene, V., Vlaminck, S., and Casselman, J.W. "Ramsay Hunt Syndrome: Pathophysiology of cochleovestibular symptoms." *Journal of Laryngology and Otology*, 116:844-848, 2002.

Sweeney, C.J., and Gilden, D.H. "Ramsay Hunt syndrome." *Journal of Neurology, Neurosurgery, and Psychiatry*, 71(2):149-154, 2001.

Zammit-Maempel, I., and Campbell, R.S. "Prolonged contrast enhancement of the inner ear on MRI in Ramsay Hunt syndrome." *British Journal of Radiology*, 68(807):334-5, 1995.

Chapter Thirty-five
Superior Semicircular Canal Dehiscence

Superior semicircular canal dehiscence is an inner ear bone abnormality. In this deformity the superior semicircular canal, the upper most canal, is not completely covered by bone. This defect apparently allows pressure changes to bring on vestibular symptoms and abnormal eye movements in some people.

The symptoms include vertigo, imbalance, unsteadiness and visual tilting or bouncing during sudden pressure changes from things like whistling, humming, bearing down, heavy lifting, and a change in the pressure of the external ear canal. Constant disequilibrium (a vague sense of unsteadiness, imbalance and/or tilting) is also common. There have been reports of one or two people also developing a hearing loss.

The diagnosis is made when the history matches, the eyes show the distinctive abnormal movements during a pressure change and the anatomical abnormality is seen on a temporal bone CT. Unfortunately not all CT scanners take good enough pictures to show it and many radiologists and ENT's don't know to look for it.

> **Technical point:** During this pressure change the eyes will show a distinctive up/down and twisting movement related to the position of the superior semicircular canal.

Treatment options include do nothing, suppress the symptoms with drugs or do surgery to plug up the abnormal opening.

References and Reading List:

Brantberg, K., Bergenius, J., Mendel, L., Witt, H., Tribukait, A., and Ygge, J. "Symptoms, findings and treatment in patients with dehiscence of the superior semicircular canal." *Acta Otolaryngologica,* 121(1):68-75, 2001.

Brantberg, K., Bergenius, J., and Tribukait, A. "Vestibular-evoked myogenic potentials in patients with dehiscence of the superior semicircular canal." *Acta Otolaryngologica, 119(6):633-40, 1999.*

Carey, J.P., Minor, L.B., and Nager, G.T. "Dehiscence or thinning of bone overlying the superior semicircular canal in a temporal bone survey." *Archives of Otolaryngology-Head and Neck Surgery,* 126(2):137-147, 2000.

Cremer, P.D., Minor, L.B., Carey, J.P., and Della Santina, C.C. "Eye movements in patients with superior canal dehiscence syndrome align with the abnormal canal." *Neurology,* 55(12):1833-1841, 2000.

Hamid, M.A. "Bilateral dehiscence of the superior semicircular canals." *Otology and Neurotology,* 22(4):567-568, 2001.

Hirvonen, T.P., Carey, J.P., Liang, C.J., and Minor, L.B. "Superior canal dehiscence: mechanisms of pressure sensitivity in a chinchilla model." *Archives of Otolaryngology-Head and Neck Surgery,* 127(11):1331-1336, 2001.

Minor, L.B. "Superior canal dehiscence syndrome." *American Journal of Otology,* 21(1):9-19, 2000.

Minor, L.B., Solomon, D., Zinreich, J.S., and Zee, D.S. "Sound- and/or pressure-induced vertigo due to bone dehiscence of the superior semicircular canal." *Archives of Otolaryngology-Head and Neck Surgery,* 124(3):249-258, 1998.

Ostrowski, V.B., Byskosh, A., and Hain, T.C. "Tullio phenomenon with dehiscence of the superior semicircular canal." *Otology and Neurotology,* 22(1):61-65, 2001.

Chapter Thirty-six
Syphilis

Syphilis, of all things, can also cause vestibular problems. Syphilis affecting hearing and balance function is generally referred to as otosyphilis. Despite the fact that a treatment exists, syphilis still flourishes around the world. It doesn't get the publicity of say, AIDS, but it continues to be a public menace because when left untreated it can create a multitude of problems all around the body.

A person can be born with it or catch it later. The symptoms of otosyphilis depend upon what stage the syphilis is in, the area infected and if a person is born with it or catches it on their own.

One in three people born with syphilis will develop vestibular symptoms. Some of these folks are as old as 60 before they have their first symptoms.

People can catch syphilis at any sexually active time during their lives and vestibular symptoms can develop at any point after they contract the infection.

In adults it commonly causes episodes of hearing loss, tinnitus, and vertigo, usually in both ears, that progresses until the hearing is gone and the vestibular function loss massive. The vertigo can be caused by sound and/or pressure. Non-ear symptoms including rash, swollen lymph nodes, and the symptoms of neurosyphilis can also occur.

This infection is diagnosed with a blood test called the FTA-ABS. Another test, the VDRL, is available but not as good at diagnosing secondary or late syphilis. The FTA-ABS tests for antibodies that have developed due to syphilis exposure but it doesn't automatically mean syphilis is the cause of the inner ear symptoms.

Antibiotic treatment with penicillin (people with a penicillin allergy may be given tetracycline) should follow the most current recommendations for the treatment of neurosyphilis from the Centers for Disease Control. The antibiotic treatment can last from two weeks to three months and may be via IV to be sure the drug gets into the spinal fluid and to the brain. Some doctors also give steroids with the antibiotic therapy.

The outcome of treatment in one study showed hearing improved in 6 people, tinnitus improved in 10 and of the 9 people in the study with vertigo, 3 were unchanged and 6 had an improvement. In three other small studies 66%, 58% and 86% of the people with vertigo improved with treatment.

At the very least, treatment should stop the progression of the damage and at its best may stop all the symptoms. Unfortunately syphilis can cause inner ear damage leading to endolymphatic hydrops which can leave people with continuing ear problems after the infection has gone.

References and Reading List:

Amenta, C.A., Dayal, V.S., Flaherty, J., and Weil, R.J. "Luetic endolymphatic hydrops: diagnosis and treatment." *American Journal of Otology*, 13(6):516-524, 1992.

Chan, Y.M., Adams, D.A., and Kerr, A.G. "Syphilitic labyrinthitis—an update." *Journal of Laryngology and Otology*, 109(8):719-725, 1995.

Fayad, J.N., and Linthicum, F.H. "Temporal bone histopathology case of the month: otosyphilis." *American Journal of Otology*, 20(2):259-60, 1999.

Gleich, L.L., Linstrom, C.J., and Kimmelman, C.P. "Otosyphilis: a diagnostic and therapeutic dilemma." *Laryngoscope*, 102(11):1255-1259, 1992.

Huang, T.S., and Lin, C.C. "Endolymphatic sac surgery for refractory luetic vertigo." *American Journal of Otology*, 12(3):184-187, 1991.

Linstrom, C.J., and Gleich, L.L. "Otosyphilis: diagnostic and therapeutic update." *Journal of Otolaryngology*, 22(6):401-408, 1993.

Nagasaki, T., Watanabe, Y., Aso, S., and Mizukoshi, K. "Electrocochleography in syphilitic hearing loss." *Acta Otolaryngologica Supplement*, 504:68-73, 1993.

Pulec, J.L. "Meniere's disease of syphilitic etiology." *Ear Nose Throat Journal*, 76(8):508-510, 512, 514, 1997.

Ruckenstein, M.J., Prasthoffer, A., Bigelow, D.C., Von Feldt, J.M., and Kolasinski, S.L. "Immunologic and serologic testing in patients with Meniere's disease." *Otology and Neurotology*, 23(4):517-521, 2002.

Smith, M.M., and Anderson, J.C. "Neurosyphilis as a cause of facial and vestibulocochlear nerve dysfunction: MR imaging features." *American Journal of Neuroradiology*, 21(9):1673-1675, 2000.

Chapter Thirty-seven
Temporal Bone Fracture

As mentioned earlier in the book the inner ear is encased in the temporal bone. If the head is struck just right this bone can be broken affecting both vestibular function and hearing and in some circumstances the facial nerve too. There are three types of breaks, longitudinal, transverse and oblique (also called mixed). Longitudinal breaks are the most common making up 70 to 90% of the total. All of these are diagnosed with a CT scan of the skull.

> **Note:** Because the temporal bone happens to be a part of the skull a doctor may refer to its fracture as a skull fracture.

Longitudinal Fracture

A longitudinal break usually damages the tympanic membrane and breaks the little middle ear bones but does not pass through the inner ear itself. This break causes hearing loss and can also cause vestibular symptoms (usually much milder than with a transverse fracture).

Treatment depends on the extent of the middle ear damage. Surgery on the ossicles and/ or the tympanic membrane may be needed, drugs may be used to suppress vertigo and stop nausea/vomiting. These can be followed by vestibular rehabilitation therapy.

Transverse Fracture

The transverse fracture is the most severe of the three types of temporal bone fracture. This fracture can run right through the inner ear and severely damage the vestibulocochlear nerve. On top of that it can rip the facial nerve causing the eyelid to be frozen open and one side of the face to droop.

If the vestibulocochlear nerve is cut completely through all hearing is lost and the flow of vestibular information to the brain is stopped, on that side. When that information flow is suddenly cut off strong vertigo and nystagmus begin along with nausea and vomiting. The first two or three days can be a blur of vertigo and vomiting for many people with drugs to suppress the vertigo and stop the vomiting needed.

The fracture will heal but the lost function will not come back. Fortunately one good inner ear is all the body needs for balance and for the vestibular reflexes to work.

Over the first days to weeks the brain readjusts and changes the way it works so movement and gravity information from only one ear can be used successfully for balance and the vestibular reflexes. This begins to occur spontaneously in most people as they look around and move their heads. Some folks will need a bit of a kick-start to get this going. The current wisdom seems to be that all people in this position can benefit from vestibular rehabilitation therapy.

Before the brain changes it's way of using the vestibular information, formally called vestibular compensation, there will be a general feeling of unsteadiness, lightheadedness, spatial disorientation and probably trouble with balance in the dark or with the eyes closed. Most people will progress to the point of both feeling and functioning in a normal way with no symptoms.

If the tear in the cochlear portion of the vestibulocochlear nerve is complete normal hearing is gone and a cochlear implant can't help. A complete one-sided loss is a problem during certain activities for obvious reasons. Whispering into that ear can't be heard, the telephone can't be answered on that side any more and conversations on the side of the dead ear will be difficult to follow. Not so obvious is that the ability to detect sound direction is lost as well. If someone yells "over here" a person with a complete one-sided loss will not immediately know where "here" is.

Oblique or Mixed Fracture

The oblique or mixed type of fracture doesn't have a typical set of problems but rather a mixture of both the longitudinal and transverse.

Complications

All three types of fractures place a person at risk for developing meningitis until the fracture mends. Other vestibular problems, including perilymphatic fistula and labyrinthine concussion, can also be caused by a traumatic fracture of the temporal bone. If one of these other vestibular problems is present their diagnosis and treatment may be difficult.

References and Reading List:

Alvi, A., and Bereliani, A. "Trauma to the temporal bone: diagnosis and management of complications." *Journal of Craniomaxillofacial Trauma,* 2(3):36-48, 1996.

Chen, J., Ji, C., Yang, C., and Liu, Z. "Temporal bone fracture and its complications." *Chinese Journal of Traumatology,* 4(2):106-109, 2001.

Darrouzet, V., Duclos, J.Y., Liguoro, D., Truilhe, Y., De Bonfils, C., and Bebear, J.P. "Management of facial paralysis resulting from temporal bone fractures: Our experience in 115 cases." *Otolaryngology-Head and Neck Surgery,* 125(1):77-84, 2001.

Swartz, J.D. "Temporal bone trauma." *Seminars in Ultrasound, CT and MR,* 22(3):219-228, 2001.

Chapter Thirty-eight
Vascular Loop Syndrome

Right off the bat I have to say this disorder is controversial. Many doctors never make this diagnosis, while others do.

This syndrome is thought to occur when a blood vessel presses on the vestibulocochlear nerve and causes inner ear symptoms. It's controversial in part because this nerve is often found to have a blood vessel pressing against it, including in people who have never had vestibular symptoms or problems of any sort.

Some of its other names are disabling positional vertigo (DPV) and cochleovestibular nerve compression syndrome.

Vascular loop syndrome can just begin out of the blue or be set into motion by trauma. Symptoms include disabling vertigo, constant tinnitus, hearing loss (in the high pitches and constant), constant disequilibrium (a vague sense of unsteadiness, imbalance and/or tilting), motion intolerance, positional vertigo, constant nausea, and perhaps even vomiting The symptoms seem worse when standing up and moving about and best when staying still in bed. The vertigo can come in waves but that isn't the most common situation. Sometimes the symptoms are worsened by vestibular suppressant drugs like meclizine or improved by low dose Valium. The symptoms are generally so bad a person can't function normally in either social functions or at work.

The diagnosis is made by the history and ruling out other possible reasons for the symptoms. An MRI or air contrast CT can be done to see if a vessel is pressing on the nerve. Some doctors also feel an auditory brainstem reflex test can pick up changes from this disorder.

Some doctors have suggested that the use of small amounts of diazepam (Valium), alprazolam (Xanax) or clonazepam (Klonopin) can suppress the symptoms. Vestibular rehabilitation therapy has also been helpful in some people. When people have symptoms that are so bad they just can't function, surgery may be suggested.

Surgery, microvascular decompression, for this disorder is a serious step because it takes place very close to the brain and isn't a sure thing by any means. At least one expert has put the chance of the vestibular symptoms improving at only 50%.

References and Reading List:
Applebaum, E.L., and Valvasori, G.E. "Auditory and vestibular system findings in patients with vascular loops in the internal auditory canal." *Annals of Otology, Rhinology, and Laryngology*, 92(112):63-69, 1984.

Bejjani, G.K., and Sekhar, L.N. "Repositioning of the vertebral artery as treatment for neurovascular compression syndromes. Technical note." *Journal of Neurosurgery*, 86(4):728-732, 1997.

Benecke, J.E., and Hitselberger, W.E. "Vertigo caused by basilar artery compression of the eighth nerve." *Laryngoscope*, 98(8 Pt 1):807-809, 1988.

Herzog, J.A., Bailey, S., and Meyer, J. "Vascular loops of the internal auditory canal: a diagnostic dilemma." *American Journal of Otology*, 18(1):26-31, 1997.

Jannetta, P.J. "Outcome after microvascular decompression for typical trigeminal neuralgia, hemifacial spasm, tinnitus, disabling positional vertigo, and glossopharyngeal neuralgia (honored guest lecture)." *Clinical Neurosurgery*, 44:331-383, 1997.

Janetta, P.J., Moller, M.B., and Moller, A.R. "Disabling positional vertigo." *New England Journal of Medicine*, 310(26):1700-1705, 1984.

Kanzaki, J., and Koyama, E. "Vascular loops in internal auditory canal as possible cause of Meniere's disease." *Auris-Nasis-Larynx*, Supplement 11:105-111, 1986.

Makins, A.E., Nikolopoulos, T.P., Ludman, C., and O'Donoghue, G.M. "Is there a correlation between vascular loops and unilateral auditory symptoms?" *Laryngoscope*, 108(11 Pt 1):1739-1742, 1998.

McCabe, B.F., and Gantz, B.J. "Vascular loop as a cause of incapacitating dizziness." *American Journal of Otology*, 10:117-120, 1989.

McCabe, B.F., and Harker, L.A. "Vascular loop as a cause of vertigo." *Annals of Otology, Rhinology, and Laryngology*, 92:542-543, 1983.

McLaughlin, M.R., Jannetta, P.J., Clyde, B.L., Subach, B.R., Comey, C.H., and Resnick, D.K. "Microvascular decompression of cranial nerves: lessons learned after 4400 operations." *Journal of Neurosurgery*, 90(1):1-8, 1999.

Meyerhoff, W.L., and Mickey, B.E. "Vascular decompression of the cochlear nerve in tinnitus sufferers." *Laryngoscope*, 98:602-604, 1988.

Moller, M.B. "Vascular compression of the eighth cranial nerve as a cause of vertigo." *Keio Journal of Medicine*, 40(3):146-150, 1991.

Okamura, T., Kurokawa, Y., Ikeda, N., Abiko, S., Ideguchi, M., Watanabe, K., and Kido, T. "Microvascular decompression for cochlear symptoms." *Journal of Neurosurgery*, 93(3):421-426, 2000.

Schwaber, M.K., and Hall, J.W. "Cochleovestibular nerve compression syndrome, I. Clinical features and audiovestibular findings." *Laryngoscope*, 102:1020-1029, 1992.

Schwaber, M.K., and Whetsell, W.O. "Cochleovestibular nerve compression syndrome. II.

Vestibular nerve histopathology and theory of pathophysiology." *Laryngoscope,* 102:1030-1036, 1992.

Wiet, R.J., Schramm, D.R., and Kazan, R.P. "The retrolabyrinthine approach and vascular loop." *Laryngoscope,* 99:1035-1040, 1989.

Chapter Thirty-nine
Vestibular Neuronitis/Neuritis

This is an inflammation of the vestibular branch of the vestibulocochlear nerve usually affecting only one ear and thought to be caused by a virus. It's the second most common vestibular disorder some ear experts see in their practice.

Note: The vestibulocochlear nerve runs from the inner ear to the brain and carries hearing and balance information.

It may also be referred to as vestibular neuritis. Vestibular neuronitis along with its sister disorder, viral labyrinthitis, are sometimes referred to as viral neurolabyrinthitis.

Sometimes vestibular neuronitis begins totally out of the blue and other times it comes within a week or two after having a cold or the flu. A person may feel a bit off for hours to days before the start of the vestibular symptoms or it might come like a bolt of lightening out of the blue.

There is no hearing loss or tinnitus with this disorder. Instead, vertigo, nausea and vomiting are the major symptoms and nystagmus can be seen as well.

This is the sort of vertigo that causes a person to lie in bed on their side hanging on to their pillow with one hand and something to vomit into in the other. Although it probably feels like forever the vertigo does begin to stop in 24 to 48 hours. It can be another 5 days before a person can get up and move about on their own. They will have trouble walking in a straight line and will probably lean to the side and have motion insensitivity for a while. It can be as many as 6 weeks before they feel fit enough to go back to work and it isn't unusual to have feelings of imbalance 6 months after the episode.

The vertigo is bad because the flow of information from the inner ear to the brain is cut off abruptly. If this damage is permanent the other ear should be able to take over in the next few weeks through vestibular compensation. It's thought that anti-vomiting and anti-vestibular drugs should be stopped as early as possible to aid in this process.

The diagnosis is an assumption because there's no way to prove that the nerve is under attack from a virus in a living person. An MRI may show a problem with the nerve but not if it's caused by a virus. Some vestibular tests show an abnormality but again not a change that can prove a virus is the cause.

Treatments in the acute phase fall into several categories:

• Grin and bear it

- Block the symptoms
- Anti-inflammatory drugs such as steroids
- Anti-viral drugs
- IV fluids if vomiting is uncontrollable

After the vertigo and vomiting slow down getting out of bed and moving around are the most important treatment. This may be done alone or with a therapist who can design a personalized vestibular rehabilitation therapy program.

Some doctors believe vestibular neuronitis can come back again and again while others don't think this is the case. There's no proof one-way or the other.

The prognosis for this disorder is usually pretty good with 50 to 75% or more going back to their lives and jobs with nothing more than a bad memory of the ordeal. Unfortunately imbalance and disequilibrium (a vague sense of unsteadiness, imbalance and/or tilting) can dog some people for years. Another vestibular disorder, BPPV, can also occur in these folks as a result of this disorder.

References and Reading List:

Davis, L.E. "Viruses and vestibular neuritis: review of human and animal studies." *Acta Otolaryngologica*, Supplement 503:70-73, 1993.

Davis, L.E., and Johnsson, L.G. "Viral infections of the inner ear: clinical, virologic, and pathologic studies in humans and animals." *American Journal of Otolaryngology*, 4(5):347-362, 1983.

Gacek, R.R., and Gacek, M.R. "Vestibular neuronitis." *American Journal of Otology, 20(4):553-554, 1999.*

Hirata, Y., Sugita, T., Gyo, K., and Yanagihara, N. "Experimental vestibular neuritis induced by herpes simplex virus." *Acta Otolaryngologica*, Supplement 503:79-81, 1993.

Hirata, T., Sekitani, T., Okinaka, Y., and Matsuda, Y. "Serovirological study of vestibular neuronitis." *Acta Otolaryngologica*, Supplement, 468:371-373, 1989.

Nadol, J.B. "Vestibular neuritis." *Otolaryngology-Head and Neck Surgery*, 112(1):162-172, 1995.

Ryu, J.H. "Vestibular neuritis: an overview using a classical case." *Acta Otolaryngologica*, Supplement 503:25-30, 1993.

Schuknecht, H.F., and Kitamura, K. "Vestibular neuritis." *Annals of Otology, Rhinology, and Laryngology*, Supplement J90(1 Pt 2):1-19, 1981.

Chapter Forty
Vertebrobasilar Insufficiency/Vertebrobasilar Occlusion

The vertebrobasilar circulatory system supplies the inner ear, vestibulocochlear nerve, vestibular nuclei of the brain and assorted brain areas with their blood supply. A partial blockage in this system is called vertebrobasilar insufficiency and a total blockage is called vertebrobasilar occlusion. When a partial or total blockage takes place all sorts of symptoms and problems are possible.

> **Technical point**: The vertebrobasilar blood supply flows through the basilar artery and then through either the anterior inferior cerebellar artery or the posterior inferior cerebellar artery. The first vessel supplies the inner ear, vestibulocochlear nerve, vestibular nuclei and some other brain areas and the second supplies the vestibular nuclei and the cerebellum of the brain.

This blood vessel system can be affected by the very same problems blood vessels in other parts of the body suffer through. Plaque can build up and slowly reduce blood flow. A blood clot or piece of debris from another part of the body can flow in and create a logjam. A vessel can even be squeezed shut by pressure.

A number of body wide conditions can cause partial or total blockage including high cholesterol (hypercholesterolemia), atherosclerosis, high blood pressure, diabetes mellitus (sugar diabetes), polycythemia (or any other condition causing the blood to thicken and clot more easily), sticky platelets, low blood pressure upon standing, cervical spondylosis and possibly, but only possibly, squishing of the vessels by turning or bending the neck.

Like a lot of other inner ear conditions, partial blockage is thought to cause momentary vertigo and hearing loss that may or may not include nausea, vomiting and nystagmus. If the partial blockage is at the beginning of the vertebrobasilar system other additional brain areas can also be affected causing symptoms like momentary loss of all vision. In some people this may occur along with little brain attacks called transient ischemic attacks (TIA).

A full blockage can create some pretty striking ear symptoms including massive hearing loss and violent vertigo. This is the sort of vertigo that causes a person to lie in bed on their side hanging on to their pillow with one hand and something to vomit into in the other. Although it probably feels like forever the vertigo does begin to stop in 24 to 48 hours. It can be another

5 days before the person can get up and move about on their own but they will have trouble walking in a straight line and probably lean to the side and have motion insensitivity for a while. It can be as long as 6 weeks before they feel good enough to get back to work.

No slam-dunk test exists to figure out if inner ear symptoms are coming from either of these conditions. A doctor will look at the history and physical examination to rule out what they can and see if there's a body wide problem to explain the symptoms. They'll also think more about this diagnosis in someone older than 65 years of age. Blood tests for cholesterol, blood sugar, thick blood, clotting too easily and sticky platelets can be done.

If an underlying problem can be found treatment will be aimed at it. For example, if cholesterol is elevated lifestyle changes such as an increase in exercise or a change in diet can be tried and if that doesn't work a cholesterol-lowering drug may be used. A daily low-dose aspirin tablet might be tried if sticky platelets are the problem. Diet change can also be tried for hypertension and if that doesn't work out medication can be added.

Vestibular suppression drugs can be used for acute attacks of vertigo and vomiting if they occur. Vestibular rehabilitation therapy exercises can help to improve balance and reduce feelings of unsteadiness when permanent damage has occurred.

The prognosis for these two problems differs quite a bit. If the problem creating the insufficiency isn't fixed or can't be fixed the hearing loss can worsen and/or become permanent. Balance function can deteriorate and symptoms increase over time as well.

If a blockage occurs and isn't reversed the hearing and balance damage are usually permanent. If this is a one sided problem the brain can readjust to only getting balance information from one side and the person can get back to normal functioning. If the opposite side is affected as well, problems can dog the person indefinitely.

References and Reading List:

Baloh, R.W. "The dizzy patient." *Postgraduate*, 105(2):161-4, 167-172, 1999.

Baloh, R.W. "Vertigo." *Lancet*, 352(9143):1841-1846, 1998.

Bruyn, G.W. "Vertigo and vertebrobasilar insufficiency. A critical comment." *Acta Otolaryngologica*, Supplement, 460:128-134, 1988.

Heidrich, H., and Bayer, O. "Symptomatology of the subclavian steal syndrome." *Angiology*, 20(7):406-413, 1969.

Hirschberg, M., and Hofferberth, B. "Calcium antagonists in an animal model of vertebrobasilar insufficiency." *Acta Otolaryngologica*, Supplement, 460:61-65, 1988.

Oosterveld, W.J. "The effectiveness of piracetam in vertigo." *Pharmacopsychiatry*, Supplement 32,1:54-60, 1999.

Taylor, C.L., Selman, W.R., and Ratcheson, R.A. "Steal affecting the central nervous system." *Neurosurgery*, 50(4):679-688; discussion 688-689, 2002.

Chapter Forty-one
Vestibulopathy

Vestibulopathy is a general term meaning disease of the vestibular area of the inner ear. Unilateral vestibulopathy refers to one inner ear, bilateral vestibulopathy to both ears.

The term can be used in one of two ways:

- As a general term referring to a specific vestibular disorder. For example, Meniere's disease could be referred to as a vestibulopathy
- To indicate that a nameless or unknown disorder is occurring in the vestibular area of the inner ear

Some doctors use this term when they know a problem is coming from the vestibular areas of the inner ear but:

- Don't know which disorder
- The symptoms don't fit any disorder

Don't assume a doctor using this generic term instead of something more specific is clueless or ignorant. It's more accurate, honest and less confusing to call it vestibulopathy when the symptoms just don't fit a specific disease pattern.

Chapter Forty-two
von Hippel-Lindau Disease

This is a genetic (inherited) disease in which some blood vessels grow abnormally into clumps called angiomas. These clumps can grow in many areas throughout the body including the endolymphatic sac of the inner ear. Sometimes a cyst also grows alongside the clump.

Although the disease was discovered in the first twenty years of the twentieth century it wasn't until 1993 that the inner ear variety was identified. Only 1 in 32,000 people has von Hippel-Lindau and as many as 11% of these might have an endolymphatic sac growth.

Hearing loss, ear ringing and vestibular symptoms are possible when it does affect the inner ear. About 2/3 of people with sac growths will have vestibular symptoms that can include vertigo, disequilibrium (a vague sense of unsteadiness, imbalance and/or tilting) a tendency to fall and nystagmus.

The affects of this disorder vary from person to person so no generalization can be made.

The blood vessel clumps can occur at the same time in other body areas as well and cause many different problems including high blood pressure, headache, vision loss and numbness. Which symptoms occur depends upon the location, the size of the clump and what the clump is pressing against.

A temporal bone MRI is the test most apt to detect endolymphatic sac involvement. DNA testing may also be done to figure out if von Hippel-Lindau disease is the culprit. CT scans and ultrasound may be used to detect clumps in other areas of the body.

Currently the only recommended treatment for the inner ear variety of angioma is surgical removal.

More information and moral support can be obtained from the von Hippel-Lindau Family Alliance. von Hippel-Lindau Family Alliance, www.vhl.org, info@vhl.org and 171 Clinton Rd., Brookline, MA 02445, 1-800-767-4847.

References and Reading List:
Ayadi, K., Mahfoudh, K.B., Khannous, M., and Mnif, J. "Lindau disease: imaging features." *American Journal of Roentgenology, 175(3):925-926, 2000.*

Choyke, P.L., Glenn, G.M., Walther, M.M., Patronas, N.J., Linehan, W.M., and Zbar, B. "von Hippel-Lindau disease: genetic, clinical, and imaging features." *Radiology,* 194(3):629-642, 1995.

Hamazaki, S., Yoshida, M., Yao, M., Nagashima, Y., Taguchi, K., Nakashima, H., and Okada, S. "Mutation of von Hippel-Lindau tumor suppressor gene in a sporadic endolymphatic sac tumor." *Human Pathology*, 32(11):1272-1276, 2001.

Inanli, S., Tutkun, A., Ozturk, O., and Ahyskaly, R. "Endolymphatic sac tumor: a case report." *Auris Nasus Larynx*, 28(3):245-248, 2001.

Kempermann, G., Neumann, H.P., and Volk, B. "Endolymphatic sac tumours." *Histopathology*, 33(1):2-10, 1998.

Luff, D.A., Simmons, M., Malik, T., Ramsden, R.T., and Reid, H. "Endolymphatic sac tumours." *Journal of Laryngology and Otology*, 116(5):398-401, 2002.

Maher, E.R., and Kaelin, W.G. "von Hippel-Lindau disease." *Medicine (Baltimore)*, 76(6):381-391, 1997.

Manski, T.J., Heffner, D.K., Glenn, G.M., Patronas, N.J., Pikus, A.T., Katz, D., Lebovics, R., Sledjeski, K., Choyke, P.L., Zbar, B., Linehan, W.M., and Oldfield, E.H. "Endolymphatic sac tumors. A source of morbid hearing loss in von Hippel-Lindau disease." *Journal of the American Medical Association*, 14:277(18):1461-1466, 1997.

Megerian, C.A., Haynes, D.S., Poe, D.S., Choo, D.I., Keriakas, T.J., and Glasscock, M.E. "Hearing preservation surgery for small endolymphatic sac tumors in patients with von Hippel-Lindau syndrome." *Otology and Neurotology*, 23(3):378-387, 2002.

Richard, S., David, P., Marsot-Dupuch, K., Giraud, S., Beroud, C., and Resche, F. "Central nervous system hemangioblastomas, endolymphatic sac tumors, and von Hippel-Lindau disease." *Neurosurgery Review*, 23(1):1-22; discussion 23-24, 2000.

Tibbs, R.E., Bowles, A.P., Raila, F.A., Fratkin, J.D., and Hutchins, J.B. "Should endolymphatic sac tumors be considered part of the von Hippel-Lindau complex? Pathology case report." *Neurosurgery*, 40(4):848-855; 1997.

Vortmeyer, A.O., Choo, D., Pack, S.D., Oldfield, E., and Zhuang, Z. "von Hippel-Lindau disease gene alterations associated with endolymphatic sac tumor." *Journal of the National Cancer Institute*, 2:89(13):970-972, 1997.

Chapter Forty-three
More

What else is there to know about vestibular disorders? In a word, lots. Just as testing and treatment are similar from one disorder to the next the affects of vestibular disorders and ways to adapt to them can be similar as well. The causes of vestibular disorders may be quite different but the symptoms and the affects of the disorder can be quite similar and studied together.

The full experience of a vestibular disorder goes well beyond a list of symptoms. Over the next few chapters vertigo, vestibular loss, imbalance, anxiety/panic, stress, fatigue and thought/memory will be covered

These chapters are then followed by three more with information about pressure, anesthesia and hormones.

Chapter Forty-four
Vestibular Loss

Signals are constantly sent from the vestibular areas of the inner ears to the brain. Lots of signals are sent, as many as 100 per millisecond, even when we're still as could be.

Once the information is in the brain it's analyzed to determine position in space and the direction of movement. Signals are then sent out to the muscles so we can move about. The brain is accustomed to getting lots of information from both ears and it likes to stick to that routine. When the routine is stopped, from any cause, there can be he- - to pay in both symptoms and problems with function.

One-sided Loss

One-sided loss can be sudden, not so sudden, total, partial, temporary and/or permanent. In general the symptoms a person has from a vestibular loss depend upon the amount of function present when the loss occurs, the amount of function lost and the speed of the loss. The strongest symptoms come from the fastest, largest losses in people who have the most remaining function. Yes, the most remaining function.

Sudden and total

The flow of vestibular information can stop suddenly and totally from problems like vestibular neuronitis, labyrinthitis, gentamicin (and other vestibulotoxic drugs), temporal bone fracture or surgery (vestibular nerve section, labyrinthectomy).

If the ear had MOST of its vestibular function up and running when the loss occurred and the loss was total there can be some pretty strong symptoms and major troubles with balance. Functional difficulties and symptoms aren't nearly so dramatic if a great deal of the vestibular function was already missing.

When vestibular function is suddenly lost, strong, even violent vertigo begins along with nystagmus (eye jerking). This vertigo is the sort that causes a person to lie in bed on their side hanging on to their pillow with one hand and something to vomit into with the other.

Balance becomes difficult because the brain is no longer getting information from both ears so it can neither analyze information nor send out signals the way it used to.

Vestibular compensation occurs solely within the brain and is a chemical process involving neurotransmitters. This term is used by the health care community to refer to the process of the brain re-wiring after a loss.

Unlike the beginning of the loss, the end is not sudden. It can feel like forever but the vertigo, vomiting and nystagmus do begin to ease off a bit in 24 to 48 hours. Luckily the brain will immediately and automatically begin to find a new way to analyze and use the information from only one ear in a process called vestibular compensation. If the brain begins its compensation process immediately and it proceeds at a normal pace a person can expect to be feeling and acting "normally" in a few weeks to a month or two.

As the compensation proceeds the vertigo lessens in intensity to the point where it might be gone when sitting or lying still but may hit again when moving the eyes, while the eyes are closed, when moving the head, or while watching a moving object. Standing or walking in the dark and on an uneven surface (like in a parking garage) will also be tough.

Sudden and partial

In a partial loss the symptoms will also depend upon how much function existed at the time of the loss and the amount of the loss. The symptoms range from mild to very strong.

Slow loss

This usually happens without a lot of fireworks. No vertigo, nystagmus, and vomiting with this one—instead there's an odd feeling of things not being right, imbalance, an unsteady feeling, bumping into things, lightheadedness and trouble moving and standing in the dark or on uneven surfaces.

This loss may occur slowly enough that the brain is able to compensate as it's happening and creating few if any symptoms.

Compensation

After a one-sided loss the brain can rearrange the way it goes about doing it's business so that one ear can provide all the information needed for balance, clear vision and the other vestibular functions. This chemical brain adjustment is also referred to as vestibular compensation or central vestibular compensation.

The best way to make sure compensation gets going is to:
* Keep the eyes open and look around, with the head still
* Move the head slowly a few times each hour, back and forth, up and down
* Take as few anti-vertigo, anti-pain, anti-vomiting/anti-nausea and sedative drugs as possible and don't drink alcohol

If the eyes feel pretty "wild" staring at an object about 18 inches to 2 feet from the face that isn't moving at all and that isn't visually busy can calm them (looking at a striped object definitely wouldn't be a good idea).

To further help compensation along some doctors will ask a physical therapist to prescribe exercises. A physical therapist with additional training and practice in vestibular rehabilitation therapy can be very helpful in putting together a program for an individual.

Most programs include general muscle strengthening and joint flexibility, head movement, eye movement, head and eye movement together, visual fixation (keeping the vision on a still object while moving the head), standing on something soft and standing or walking with the eyes closed. These steps are aimed at forcing the brain to deal with all the different types of information it encounters. Some therapists also use a computerized machine to help in re-learning and readjusting balance.

What can cause symptoms and functional difficulties to persist? A failure to compensate and/or not relying enough on the remaining vestibular function can cause problems to remain.

When balance information from an ear is lost the brain does two things, compensation and sensory substitution. Sensory substitution means the brain will try to use vision and proprioception (collection and use of information about the length and motion of muscles and joints by nerves in the muscles, tendons, joints, ligaments and connective tissue that figures out body position, movement and gravity) for balance until it sorts out how to use the vestibular information from only one ear.

Once compensation begins the brain should go back to using all three senses for balance: vestibular, vision and proprioception. Any situation without visual or proprioceptive information or with confusing information can cause symptoms and balance problems. Examples include: Watching moving objects, walking on soft surfaces, walking in fluorescent lighting.

A vestibular rehabilitation program has a pretty good shot at helping with this problem. A therapist can suggest exercises that will force the brain to use vestibular information more while reducing the use of vision and proprioception.

Compensation can be slowed or stopped if there's a problem in the opposite ear, a brain injury or disorder, if a person doesn't open their eyes and look around enough, keeps their head too still, doesn't move their head and eyes together, doesn't get out of bed within a day or two, has fatigue, other illnesses, muscle weakness, or if taking pain killing drugs, alcohol, tranquilizers, sedatives, anti-vertigo drugs or anti-vomiting/anti-nausea drugs.

If compensation isn't complete any number of symptoms and/or problems can occur including: vertigo with the eyes closed, vertigo during head movement, vertigo watching moving objects, nystagmus with the eyes closed; an unsteady/unbalanced feeling, unsteady balance, constant feeling of movement, unsteadiness, light headedness, heavy headedness, and bumping into things otherwise known as disequilibrium.

Compensation isn't permanent. It can fluctuate quite a bit and be temporarily undone (decompensation) by all the things that can hold up or interfere with achieving compensation in the first place. Luckily the symptoms are generally mild and compensation comes back quickly once the cause is gone, i.e. the cold goes away, the drug passes out of the system, etc.

Two-sided Loss

Information is constantly collected from both ears and sent on to the brain where it's analyzed to figure out position in space and movement direction. The brain uses this information to send out movement signals that help in moving about safely and seeing clearly. If this ability is lost a dramatic, life-altering (some might even say life destroying) change occurs.

Just like the one-sided type, two-sided loss also comes in several ways including sudden, not so sudden, total, partial, temporary, permanent, equal and unequal. These can occur in many different combinations.

In general the symptoms from this loss depend upon the amount of function present when the loss occurred, the amount of the loss, the speed of the loss and if the loss was nearly equal between the two ears.

The faster the loss, the larger the loss, the more function left at the time of the loss and the more unequal the signals from the two ears, the greater the symptoms and problems with function.

A two-sided loss can occur out of the blue for no apparent reason, from the use of IV gentamicin and other aminoglycoside antibiotics and possibly from an autoimmune reaction. Thankfully a sudden two-sided loss in not very common.

Sudden, total, two-sided loss

If the ear had MOST of it's vestibular function at the time of the loss, the loss was total or pretty darn close, and if the loss is equal in the two ears, there won't be violent vertigo and nystagmus like in the sudden, one-sided variety. Instead there will be a very serious loss of balance ability along with bouncing and/or blurry vision during head movement (oscillopsia). A feeling of unreality, lightheadedness, fear, and anxiety can occur along with general incoordination, difficulty with short-term memory, stiff neck, headache, fatigue and trouble with thinking.

Balance is usually impossible immediately following a sudden, total loss. Vision will appear to bounce and blur as well. Why? Because without vestibular information the brain can no longer send out the right muscle movement signals for either balance or clear vision.

The brain immediately and automatically tries to find a new way to analyze and use whatever vestibular information is available, and also use the other balance senses, vision and proprioception.

When little or no vestibular function is left, compensation won't occur. The brain must then rely solely on sensory substitution, a switch from using a combination of three senses; vestibular, visual and muscle/joint pressure sense (proprioception), to using a combination of only, two, vision and proprioception.

Balance can be done with only these two senses but this skill takes time to develop fully—as long as two years even with proper guidance from a trained and experienced therapist. More time will be required if going it alone.

This switch makes balance an almost conscious task and may be the reason that fatigue, short term memory loss and thought are problems. It's like the brain is spending its time, energy and storage space on balance instead of other things.

Balance through sensory substitution isn't nearly as good as normal balance using the three senses. When three sensory systems are used there's more back-up and the brain has more information to rely on. With only two sensory systems sending information to the brain there's lots more room for problems and misinterpretation.

Vision more easily tricks the brain into thinking movement's occurring when it isn't. In any situation where vision can't be used (like total darkness) the brain is down to only one source of information and balance can't take place. Falls will occur easily when closing the eyes or if trying to stand or move about in the dark.

When proprioception isn't fully available there can be problems as well. This can happen, for example, when walking in beach sand or on a heavily padded carpet or in a person with a disease like multiple sclerosis or long time diabetes mellitus that can decrease joint/muscle pressure sense in the legs and feet.

Sadly there's no back-up system for the vestibulocular reflex. There's little chance vision will naturally return to normal after a permanent, total, two-sided loss. Some degree of visual bouncing and blurring are going to stay.

Sudden, partial, two-sided loss

In a partial two-sided loss the symptoms depend upon how much function existed at the time of the loss, the amount of the loss and if the losses in the two ears are equal or nearly so.

If the loss is equal between the ears but not large, a person might not be aware it's happened. On the other hand if the loss is a bit bigger, a person can have just as many symptoms and changes to their life as someone with a total loss.

The amount of long-term disability from a partial two-sided loss is impossible to predict. A good program of vestibular rehabilitation therapy might go a long way in helping both sensory substitution and vestibular compensation, if there's enough vestibular function left to undergo compensation.

Slow loss

If the loss is slow enough the brain may be able to compensate as it's happening so a person might not even be aware it's happening, at first. A compensated brain is a happy brain and a happy brain doesn't create symptoms.

As the loss increases a person may slowly realize they are having both problems with balance and vision. If the loss becomes complete or nearly so, the long-term problems will be very similar to those of someone who suffered a sudden, total loss.

Unequal bilateral loss

A slow, two-sided loss that's unequal may not be felt until so much has been lost that balance and vision are affected quite a bit.

On the other hand a rapid, unequal loss can bring on the same sort of vertigo, nystagmus and vomiting that a sudden unilateral loss can cause.

The long-term outcome depends on how much was lost on both sides. If enough vestibular function is left things can get back to normal or something close to it. If vestibular compensation can't be done the outcome will be similar to the sudden, total, equal variety covered at the beginning of this chapter.

Fluctuating Function

Constant fluctuation in the amount and type of information sent from the ear to the brain is a difficult problem. This can't be said enough: a brain needs constant and consistent information equally, from both ears. Without this a person will be a very unhappy camper with lots of symptoms and problems.

From a symptom point of view this may be the most difficult of the vestibular loss situations to deal with. The brain is constantly searching for the right way to deal with the ear information but never quite gets there—or if it does the situation changes yet again and its back to square one. It's kind of like trying to hit a moving target—much more difficult then aiming for one that's dead still.

One general principle in neurotology is that a constantly changing condition is more difficult to deal with than a steady or "stable" loss. It's both harder to live with and more difficult to treat.

Fluctuations in function come in a lot of ways. They can be small, making people feel a bit off much of the time and never quite "normal" or they can be large causing violent vertigo, nystagmus and even vomiting or anything in between. Fluctuations can also occur for short periods of time followed by complete remission and compensation or they can be pretty constant. The more constant and/or the greater the amount of fluctuation, the bigger the symptoms and problems.

There is no specific symptom pattern for this problem. One person might feel like something just isn't right and another might feel like they are in a boat constantly rocking in the ocean while someone else could go from one episode to another of violent vertigo.

Some people have a feeling of constant movement that's at odds with the information the brain is getting from both the eyes and the pressure sense in the muscles and joints leaving them feeling seasick and exhausted most of the time.

Many symptoms are possible: headache, nausea, loss of appetite, light headedness, heavy headedness, feeling of floating or swimming, imbalance, stumbling around, banging into things, never feeling "right," fatigue, increased symptoms with head movement, eye movement or while watching something that's moving, panic/anxiety episodes, blurred vision, and sensitivity to fluorescent lights

One of the problems with fluctuating function is that it doesn't belong to just one vestibular disorder, it can happen with many of them so its presence may not be all that helpful in finding a diagnosis. Meniere's disease, endolymphatic hydrops, perilymphatic hydrops, migraine, and extreme cases of benign paroxysmal positional vertigo can all cause fluctuating function and a lot of misery.

When the symptoms are constant and no major attacks of spontaneous, violent vertigo, are occurring there's a chance the problem isn't fluctuating function but instead a problem with vestibular compensation. About the only way to sort this out is to try vestibular rehabilitation therapy with an experienced therapist and see if it helps.

If the underlying problem can't be fixed, stopped or slowed down, if vestibular rehabilitation therapy with a therapist educated and experienced in vestibular rehabilitation doesn't work and you are miserable and unable to function a doctor may offer drugs to suppress the symptoms or surgery to destroy the offending inner ear or nerve (when only one ear is at fault and it can be identified for sure).

Which treatment a doctor offers or if they offer anything at all will depend on what they think is wrong, their belief system about the vestibular illness and the treatments available, how much suffering is occurring, how verbal a person is about their suffering, what treatments are available in their geographic area, and their insurance coverage.

References and Reading List:

Baloh, R.W., and Halmagyi, G.M. *Disorders of the Vestibular System.* New York: Oxford University Press, 1996.

Curthoys, I.S., and Halmagyi, G.M. "Vestibular compensation." *Advances in Otorhinolaryngology,* 55:82-110, 1999.

Shepard, N.T., and Telian, S.A. *Practical Management of the Balance Disorder Patient.* San Diego: Singular Publishing Group, Inc. 1996.

Chapter Forty-five
Vertigo

Vertigo is the sense of movement that isn't happening or the misinterpretation of movement that is. Spinning, dropping, falling, floating, bouncing, or swimming sensations are all vertigo when a person isn't actually spinning, dropping, falling, floating, etc. The feeling of moving fast when actually moving slowly is also vertigo.

Vertigo can occur once or twice and go away forever or might last weeks, months or even years. It can come in episodes or attacks or be fairly constant. Attacks can come out of the blue; directly from activities like eye movement, head movement or watching moving objects; or could come from what a person is eating or even from a barometric pressure change.

The vertigo can be mild enough for a person to go on with their usual activities or be so violent they can't even get out of bed. It can occur alone or along with other symptoms like eye jerking, nausea, and vomiting.

Problems within the inner ear, vestibulocochlear nerve or the brain can cause vertigo if function is fluctuating or has been lost. It also can occur when the brain isn't able to readjust (chemically compensate) after a vestibular loss. Unfortunately why it's happening and exactly where it's coming from, even which ear or vestibulocochlear nerve is affected, can't always be determined.

As a person looks for a diagnosis, cure or treatment they need to shoulder the responsibility for dealing with the minute-to-minute reality of vertigo. It's unpleasant but there are some things a person can do to cope.

Coping With Vertigo
Study the vertigo

Spend time thinking about the vertigo and studying it. When does it occur? What does it feel like? Are there any other symptoms? How long does it go on? What seems to cause it? Does anything help?

To aid in accurately describing and discussing the vertigo with a health care professional keep an activity and symptom diary. Jot down all your activities throughout the day, when you get up, when you eat, drive, work, etc, when and what's eaten, medications taken, allergen levels (mold, pollen, etc), and barometric pressure (reported on the local news or in the newspaper). Whenever vertigo or other symptoms occur describe them in the diary.

Violent attacks

If suffering from violent attacks carry a laminated card with your name, address, several emergency contact numbers, your doctor's number and an explanation of your disorder to assist in getting help. Print or write this information on a business card sized piece of paper, laminate it and carry it in your wallet.

If experiencing incapacitating attacks of vertigo without warning DO NOT DRIVE, period. In addition to the possibility of hurting yourself other people could be injured, even killed. Instead use public transport, taxis and rides from neighbors, friends and relatives. Relatives, friends and neighbors in a person's life need to know about the condition so they understand the situation and can help when needed.

Preparation, both at home and on the go, is crucial in dealing with disabling attacks of vertigo. Know what to do, have plans in place for different situations that might arise and keep the right supplies close at hand.

Parents of young children should have a plan for picking the kids up from school when they are unable. A small child also needs reassurance that Mommy or Daddy may get sick once in a while but they will be well taken care of.

During a short attack of violent vertigo the movement sensation can sometimes be overcome by laying still and staring very hard at a stationary object about 18 inches from the face. If staring doesn't work out the next best thing is to keep the eyes shut and the head rigid while laying on something firm and still. Trying to focus ones thoughts on something besides the vertigo, anything other than the vertigo, like a schedule, math problem, favorite book or story, future plans, or prayer can help the time pass.

Medication can dull the vertigo and/or the nausea and vomiting in many people. This must be discussed with the ear specialist ahead of time so the correct medication can be prescribed and kept on hand. Since it usually won't be as effective once an attack is in full swing take medication as early as possible. Store prescribed medication where it won't get too cold, too hot or too damp but is handy.

Have a vertigo kit with comfort and emergency items at home, in the car and at work.
Home or work vertigo kit:

- Basin or bowl
- Small bottled water
- Breath mint or spray, mouthwash
- Peppermint or ginger candies
- Garbage bags
- Adult diapers
- Baby or handiwipes
- Sheet or emergency foil cover for warmth and privacy
- Clean change of clothing including underwear

Car vertigo kit can include:

- Garbage bags
- Small bottled water
- Canned beverage
- Breath mint or spray
- Peppermint or ginger candies
- Adult diapers

- Baby or handiwipes
- A sheet or emergency foil cover for warmth and privacy, in a cold climate a sleeping bag
- Cell phone (mobile phone) with emergency contacts
- Medic alert medallion with emergency contact numbers
- Pillow (small, compressible types are available wherever camping supplies are sold)
- Waterless hand cleaner
- Washcloth/towel

After an attack of violent vertigo it's fine to sleep for several hours or the rest of the day but don't spend several days in bed waiting for the feeling of imbalance to leave on its own. Walking around in a normal way with eyes open and head moving helps the body go through it's natural recovery process and gets you back on track most quickly.

Since it's hard to know how soon and how hard to push this should be discussed with an inner ear specialist or physical therapist thoroughly familiar with vestibular disorders and a person's specific situation. The waters may need to be tested quite a few times to figure out how to proceed after an attack. It may require experimentation and pushing the envelope at times.

Because an attack of violent vertigo is usually miserable, not life threatening, many people just ride it out in the comfort and privacy of their own home taking prescribed medication as needed.

If the vomiting and diarrhea go on long enough during an attack serious dehydration can occur. Most people become quite dehydrated if vomiting goes on for more than 12 to 24 hours and IV fluid replacement in a hospital may become necessary. When to get emergency help should be discussed with the ear specialist in advance.

Long lasting vertigo

If vertigo is constant but not violent lying rigidly in bed staring at something stationary isn't a good idea. Instead you must move around and carry on with your life to the best of your ability and as safely as possible.

Recovery and/or chemical compensation can be delayed or possibly even prevented by staying still and stopping all activities that bring on or worsen symptoms. Taking symptom-blocking drugs can do the same.

A doctor won't have the time to lead a person through all aspects of their life with vestibular disease but a doctor educated and experienced in vestibular disorders should provide general guidelines and medical support such as suggesting treatments and writing necessary prescriptions. A doctor unable or unwilling to discuss these issues may not be the best one to see on a long-term basis.

Provoked Vertigo

This is vertigo brought on by activities like moving the eyes, watching something that's moving, moving the head or looking at something that's visually busy, like stripes or a computer screen.

Do not RIGIDLY stop doing all the things that bring on vertigo unless it creates a dangerous situation or a specialist has advised it. Instead go about daily activities as normally as possible.

Vestibular rehabilitation therapy helps many people with provoked vertigo. If the provoked vertigo comes between closely spaced attacks of Meniere's disease (i.e. less than 3-4 weeks) vestibular rehabilitation therapy may be less effective.

If provoked vertigo continues after months of treatment, a person is sick from it all the time and their otologist confirms they can't do anything further the next step may be to stop doing the things causing it.

Try to figure out the exact thing causing the vertigo and stop only that. For example if moving the head rapidly to the left is a problem stop that, not all head movement.

Avoidance

Avoiding activities that bring on or worsen vertigo isn't the way to handle vertigo when it first starts. Not only does a reduction in activities prevent a person from getting better, it might just make them worse.

If everything thing has been tried, if diet, diuretics, anti-migraine drugs, vestibular rehabilitation therapy and all the rest have failed and symptoms are causing misery and the inability to carry on in life the only options left may be symptom blocking drugs and avoidance of anything making the symptoms worse.

Whether a person should depend solely upon avoidance and/or drugs for symptom control is a very personal decision that shouldn't be made unless there just isn't any other way to proceed. This decision should be made in close consultation with a doctor trained and experienced in vestibular disorders. A second or even third opinion from an ear specialist would be best before using symptom suppressors and avoidance as the only method for coping with vestibular symptoms.

Someone with more or less constant symptoms might benefit from vestibular rehabilitation therapy. If this treatment hasn't been suggested ask about it.

If avoidance is the only option left these ideas might help:

- If you don't get out of the house much invite people over to your place.
- Remain in contact with friends via telephone.
- Join computer groups to explore hobbies and interests.

Reading

- Use a ruler under each sentence being read to keep your eyes on the right spot
- Try the large print books or the talking books from the library for pleasure reading

TV/movie viewing

- Don't watch TV in a dark room
- Use a smaller screen so the front and side walls can be seen while watching the TV
- Sit back far enough at the movie theater to see the sidewalls in addition to the screen
- Don't go to 3D or Imax movies

Shopping

- When going to the supermarket use a cart to help with balance
- Shop from catalogs or online
- Use your supermarkets shopping service if they offer one

Vision

- A smaller computer screen or a laptop screen may cause fewer visual symptoms
- Avoid places with fluorescent lighting, strobe lights or other flickering lighting
- Progressive or bifocal glasses may increase symptoms. This can be overcome by using one for distance, one for close work and another for the computer.
- Stay away from noisy situations like basketball games and concerts
- Don't move your head while already moving in one direction. In other words if riding in the car keep your head against the headrest and pointed forward.

Technical note: Moving the head simultaneously in two different planes is the coriolis effect.

Sum Up

Because vertigo can be caused by a number of things there are many ways to deal with it. Avoiding situations that seem to bring it on or make it worse isn't the best way to deal with it but in some cases may become the only way.

Next

Imbalance is covered in the next chapter.

References and Reading List

Beidel, D.C., and Horak, F.B. "Behavior therapy for vestibular rehabilitation." *Journal of Anxiety Disorders*, 15:121-130, 2001.

Bronstein, A. "Underrated neuro-otological symptoms: Hoffman and Brookler 1978 revisited." *British Medical Bulletin*, 63:213-221, 2002.

Yardley, L., and Redfern, M.S. "Psychological factors influencing recovery from balance disorders." *Journal of Anxiety Disorders*, 15:107-119, 2001.

Chapter Forty-six
Imbalance

A person can feel imbalance or have imbalance. One can feel imbalanced without being imbalanced or have imbalance without feeling imbalance or they can occur together.

Feeling of Imbalance
The feeling of imbalance without actually having poor balance isn't physically harmful, at first. Unfortunately over time a person may stop their normal activities due to fear and a lack of confidence in the ability to balance, not because they are physically unable.

Reducing activities may feel good at first but can be a problem over the long haul. It reinforces the idea that activities can't be done and this in turn can lead to the inability to get them done. Good balance requires joint flexibility, muscle strength and both practice and experience with all the activities of life. Activities must be done over and over to maintain good balance. As the saying goes, "use it or lose it."

The fear can be controlled or overcome by slowly increasing activities requiring balance to learn they really can be done. A person can do this on his or her own, with a general physical training program or in a very structured way with a physical therapist or even a psychological counselor.

Having Imbalance
Having imbalance obviously can cause physical harm from falls and running into things. In addition it can create fear and lack of confidence in the ability to get around which over time leads to even more imbalance. Coping is aimed at safety, full use of one's remaining abilities and, when needed, reorganizing the way balance is done.

Safety
Safety comes first when having imbalance.
Make sure you have:

- Adequate lighting, particularly around steps and on uneven or sloping areas
- Night lights
- Well fitting, flat shoes with nonskid bottoms that make good contact with the ground
- Non-skid covering in the bathtub/shower

And that you:

- Remove obstacles from in and around the house
- Remove throw rugs
- Don't walk on floors that are wet or slippery
- Don't walk on ice
- Don't pilot an aircraft
- Don't drive when feeling ill or spatially disoriented, if having attacks of vertigo without warning or if too sleepy or fatigued
- Be very careful with new glasses until used to them
- Take care when walking on uneven or sloping ground
- Don't climb ladders, trees, etc
- Don't use a chain saw or other dangerous power tool
- Shower very carefully. Use tearless shampoo and keep the eyes open if standing in the shower otherwise sit in the tub or on a shower chair and use a showerhead with an extension.

Using what you have to the fullest
Vision

- Have yearly eye exams
- Always wear the correct glass prescription
- Use anti-glare coating on the glasses
- Avoid fluorescent and other lights that flicker
- Talk to your doctor about the safety of bifocal or progressive lenses if glasses are needed for both distance and reading
- Contact lenses may create less visual distortion

In general:

- Get plenty of rest
- Exercise to strengthen muscles and keep joints flexible (Can't exercise in the standing position? Use a chair or bed or even the floor but work on joint flexibility and muscle strength each day.)
- Wear shoes that allow the feet to feel the ground or floor completely (a few doctors recommend bare feet but the down side to this suggestion is the potential for injuring the feet)
- Use your hands and arms to help figure out your position in space. Touching something with as little as a finger, when you can't see, may provide enough information to prevent falling.

Reorganizing Balance
As mentioned earlier in the book the three sensory systems involved in balance are vestibular function, vision and proprioception. A physical therapist educated and experienced in vestibular

rehabilitation therapy can set up an individual program to get the most out of each of these balance senses.

Sum Up
Both feeling imbalance and having imbalance can lead to difficulty in all aspects of life. Coping is aimed at the full use of one's abilities, safety, and reorganizing the way balance is done.

Next
Tinnitus and hearing loss are covered in the next chapter.

References and Reading List:

Beidel, D.C., and Horak, F.B. "Behavior therapy for vestibular rehabilitation." *Journal of Anxiety Disorders,* 15:121-130, 2001.

Jeka, J.J., and Lackner, K.R. "Fingertip contact influences human postural control." *Experimental Brain Research,* 100:495-502, 1994.

Yardley, L. "Overview of psychologic effects of chronic dizziness and balance disorders." *Otolaryngologic Clinics of North America,* 33(3):603-616, 2000.

Yardley, L., Britten, J., Lear, S., and Bird, J. "Relationship between balance system function and agoraphobic avoidance." *Behavior Research Therapy,* 33:435-439, 1995.

Yardley, L., Britten, J., Lear, S., and Bird, J. "Relationship between balance system function and agoraphobic avoidance." *Behavior Research Therapy,* 33:435-439, 1995.

Chapter Forty-seven
Tinnitus and Hearing Loss

In some vestibular disorders hearing symptoms can also occur. The two most common symptoms are tinnitus and hearing loss.

Tinnitus

Tinnitus is the medical term for ringing in the ears or head noises. Why it occurs isn't well understood. It can be constant or on and off, loud or soft, high pitched or low pitched, a mild problem or totally distracting, even disabling.

Some levels of tinnitus can be overcome by just not thinking about it. Other levels of tinnitus might be helped by listening to noise that doesn't change in loudness or pitch like the noise made by a fan. More high tech ear help is also available from hearing professionals with both tinnitus maskers and tinnitus retraining therapy.

The tinnitus masker constantly makes noise to help cover up the tinnitus. Tinnitus retraining therapy is newer and aimed at the way the brain processes sound. The chance of success for this treatment is higher when done under the supervision of a professional well trained and experienced in the treatment.

Biofeedback, counseling and medications are also available.

Some drugs, like caffeine and aspirin, can increase the tinnitus. Stop drinking soda and other beverages containing caffeine for a week to see what affect that has on the noise level. If the tinnitus improves while off the caffeine, it can be permanently removed from the diet. There are decaffeinated versions of nearly all caffeine-containing beverages.

Aspirin problems are more common when the drug is taken in large amounts. Which drugs to avoid, if any, should be discussed with both the ear specialist and PCP to determine the best approach in a particular situation.

The American Tinnitus Association has information about tinnitus as well as some support services. ATA, P.O. Box 5, Portland, OR 92707-0005, (800) 634-8978, www.ata.org

Hearing Loss

A hearing loss can be partial or total and one-sided or two-sided. The person suffering it may choose to just live with it. They may also seek treatment and devices to get their life back to where it was. A certified audiologist, CCC-A, can help in determining what devices and equipment might be of help and will be able to make referrals to resources for the deaf and hard of hearing.

There are a great many devices for the deaf and hearing impaired. The best device for a person will depend upon:

- The type of loss
- If it's on one or both sides
- How motivated a person is
- How much rehabilitation work a person is willing to do
- Insurance coverage
- Finances
- What will work best for their family, friends and coworkers

It doesn't take a lot of imagination to understand that someone with a large hearing loss in both ears will have a great many difficulties continuing in their lives as they were. The problems faced by someone with a one-sided loss may not be so obvious and can be hard for family, friends, co-workers etc. to understand and deal with. Someone with a partial loss may seem normal one minute and impaired the next. People around them need to know they aren't engaging in selective hearing and that what they can hear will depend upon what ear is being spoken to and the level of background noise. That someone with good hearing in only one ear won't be able to figure out which direction sound is coming from.

There are many support groups and organizations for the hard or hearing and deaf including Self-Help for Hard of Hearing People at 7910 Woodmont Avenue, Suite 1200 Bethesda, Maryland, 20814, TTY 301-657-2249, www.shhh.org

Sum Up

Hearing symptoms can occur in some vestibular disorders. In addition to the groups mentioned above there are a number of self-help books available covering tinnitus, hearing loss and deafness.

Next
Anxiety, panic and fear are covered next.

Chapter Forty-eight
Anxiety, Panic and Fear

It's not unusual for someone with a vestibular disorder to have fear, anxiety or even panic. Dizziness and anxiety have been linked together for centuries. Recent studies have also shown that as a group, people with dizziness have more anxiety than people with other ear disorders and people with an anxiety disorder diagnosis, as a group, are at higher risk for abnormal vestibular tests. It's recognized as enough of a problem that a special medical meeting was held and one entire issue of the *Journal of Anxiety Disorders*, during 2001, was devoted to the relationship.

Feeling fear
The physical sensations we have when fearful, anxious or panicked come from the autonomic nervous system (ANS), the part of the nervous system using adrenaline and handling physical response to fear.

If a person walking down the street is confronted with a snarling pit bull their brain sends out signals to help in either fighting it out with the dog or running away as fast as their legs can carry them. This is known as the fight or flight response.

During a fight or flight response the ANS sends out signals throughout the body to speed up heart rate, increase blood pressure, increase the rate and depth of breathing and to dilate some blood vessels and constrict others. All these changes work to move blood, and the oxygen it carries, to the places that will help a person hit the ground running during the period of danger. This chain of events can help avoid a confrontation with danger or produce extra strength to deal with it.

Bad Fear
Unfortunately the fight or flight response can go on when there isn't a threat to physical wellbeing. In addition to being uncomfortable, fear, anxiety and the fight or flight response can change behavior. They may cause a person to not only avoid the fear but also anything related to it. This urge to avoid can be so strong a person may not leave home without someone at their side, if they leave home at all.

In addition to its mental impact the prolonged stress of a fight of flight response has been associated with a number of physical ailments such as heart disease.

A flight or flight response can come from real danger (like being chased by a bear), when the mind has blown a real fear a bit out of proportion, out of the blue (like in panic disorder) or directly from the vestibular system.

Why Dizziness and Anxiety?

The exact relationship between vestibular function and fear, anxiety and panic isn't totally understood. It does seem that dizziness can cause anxiety, anxiety can cause dizziness and both may be caused at the same time by the same thing (but not cause each other). A lot of combinations like dizziness causing anxiety that in turn causes dizziness, or anxiety that causes dizziness that goes on to cause more anxiety are also possible.

Basic science research has found that the vestibular areas of the inner ear and the areas of the brain regulating the autonomic nervous system (ANS) are linked with nerves. This nerve link allows for instant sharing of balance information with the ANS.

Since this physical link exists, it seems logical to think the information from the vestibular system may stimulate the ANS and cause symptoms directly, with no thought involved. Research continues into this relationship between anxiety/panic and the vestibular system.

Types of Fear

Fear comes in many forms at many times and has many names. Fear of a medical disorder and the disruption and uncertainty it can bring to life isn't irrational or automatically bad, particularly if a person uses it in a positive way. Some fears people with vestibular disorders have are:

- Deafness
- Embarrassment
- Falling
- Homelessness
- Injury
- Isolation
- Loneliness
- Loss of communication ability
- Loss of driving license
- Loss of independence
- Loss of job
- Loss of respect
- Not being believed

Unfortunately fear can get out of hand and produce abnormal thought patterns or behavior like that seen with a phobia, generalized anxiety disorder and/or panic disorder.

Phobia

Strong fear of a single object or situation that isn't in fact physically threatening or dangerous is considered abnormal and called a phobia. Fear of heights, acrophobia, and fear of leaving home or being someplace without an easy escape route (agoraphobia) are two examples of phobias.

Generalized anxiety disorder

This disorder includes constant worry over trivial matters, trouble sleeping, being irritable, having fatigue and being a bit wound up and restless along with anticipating the worst when thinking about the situations life presents.

Panic disorder

To meet the criteria for a diagnosis of panic disorder there must be at least two attacks, out of the blue, with at least four symptoms from the list below. Attacks with fewer than four symptoms are sometimes called limited symptom attacks.

- Chest pain
- Choking or smothering sensations
- Faintness
- Fear of losing control, dying or going crazy
- Feeling of unreality
- Feeling unsteady
- Hot or cold flashes
- Nausea or stomach pains
- Numbness or tingling
- Rapid heart beat
- Shortness of breath
- Sweating
- Trembling or shaking

Panic disorder is diagnosed in twice as many women as men. Depression also can develop in as many as 60% of people with panic disorder. It's also not unusual for agoraphobia to occur in someone with panic disorder.

Because hyperthyroidism, hypoglycemia, and hyperparathyroidism can cause similar symptoms they must be considered and ruled out.

Nobody really knows for sure why panic attacks occur but there are a number of theories falling into two groups, the biological and the psychological. The biological theories include genetics, faulty chemicals, brain malfunction and a problem with metabolism. The psychological theories include the mind misinterpreting a sensation, a conditioned response, unresolved issues of separation and the Freudian thought that it has something to do with undischarged sexual energy.

Kids and Anxiety

Younger children won't be able to tell anyone they're anxious, fearful or having panic. What may happen instead is a change in the way they act. They may seem tense or become upset easily and may want to hear from a parent that they're OK. Children may also become quiet, not want to participate in activities, might sweat abnormally and possibly experience stomachache and cramps.

Coping

Obviously getting rid of the vestibular disorder that might be causing the fear, anxiety or panic type symptoms would be best but that won't always be possible. A person may need to find a way to live on with the symptoms of a vestibular disorder.

Part of living on is dealing with fear rather than avoiding it. It's easier to figure out what to do about your fear when it's fully understood. This means the fear must be uncovered and a hard look taken at it.

Take for example the fear of losing a job. First, is it a reasonable fear? Job loss doesn't happen real often but it can, particularly when someone is forced to call out sick a lot and can't perform well at work. This fear can not only be reasonable, it can also be a wake up call to start actively working at keeping a job or looking for one that is a better fit.

A job loss might be avoided by talking to an employer or boss about limitations and trying to work out reasonable accommodation. Another approach is to work hard at finding and using strengths to become indispensable at a job. Look at this fear of job loss fully. What part of losing a job would be a problem? Loss of money? Creativity? Boredom?

Once the different parts of a fear are identified they can be dealt with one at a time. Different ideas for making or keeping more money can be considered. If unable to work disability can be applied for.

Work can be a big outlet for the creative juices flowing in all of us. Creativity can be replaced and boredom avoided, at least to some degree, by lots of different activities.

Seeking Help

If you come to the conclusion that your fear, anxiety or panic aren't warranted, you're having them out of all proportion to your situation, or are having difficulty going it alone, look for help in working through the problem.

A counselor, therapist or psychiatrist with vestibular training who will work with both you and your ear specialist would be your best choice for help. Unfortunately there are very few mental health professionals trained and experienced in vestibular disorders. Most people will have to rely upon someone without this experience.

Other strategies that different people have found helpful include talking with clergymen, telephone contact with other people with similar vestibular problems, meeting people on the Internet who have similar problems or joining a support group.

A support group can show a person how real their illness is and that they aren't alone. Acceptance, understanding, comradeship, sharing, and knowledge can all come from a support group. On the down side support group members can supply misinformation and bad advice and a support group can get between a person and their "real life" including their doctor. Don't assume your doctor will be thrilled by a patient who knows a lot about their illness or socializes with other people who have the same disorder, they may not be.

Using a support group (that meets in person or over the Internet) as an addition to a full life, during times of crisis or for additional information is fine. Using it to hide away from the world isn't. Don't live solely through your computer or meet only with people who have your disorder and wall yourself off from family and the people you know.

Treatments

There are both therapy and drug treatments for fear, anxiety and panic.

Therapy

Counselors can use any one of a number of treatment approaches aimed at thought and/or behavior including:

- Cognitive restructuring consisting of identifying and helping errors in thought that lead to untrue beliefs that start off anxiety, make it worse or keep it going longer.
- Cognitive behavioral therapy that includes cognitive restructuring, breathing retraining, fear exposure and panic monitoring.
- Relaxation training teaching techniques such as selective muscle relaxation to reverse the physical effects of the fight or flight response.

- Modeling or teaching the proper coping techniques are taught so they can be practiced and then used under supervision.
- Desensitization is gradually being exposed to the feared thing or situation with guidance and support.
- Flooding or the rapid, total exposure to the feared thing or situation is done with guidance and support.

Drugs

Drugs of the benzodiazepine drug family, including Valium, are commonly used for short periods of time for attacks of anxiety. Unfortunately long term use of these drugs is a problem because they can be addictive.

Antidepressants are used for long-term treatment of anxiety and panic and aren't addictive. They are taken to prevent anxiety and attacks of panic, not to treat attacks while they are occurring since the drugs must be taken for weeks before they are effective.

Sum Up

Fear, anxiety and panic can occur with dizziness and vestibular disorders. A number of treatments are available to help if these are interfering with life.

More information and support:

American Psychiatric Association
1400 K Street N.W.
Washington, DC 20005
202-682-6000
www.psych.org

Anxiety Disorders Association of America
11900 Parklawn Drive, Suite 100 Rockville, MD. 20852-2624
301-231-9350
www.adaa.org

National Institute of Mental Health
Information Resources and Inquiries Branch
5600 Fishers Lane, Room 7C-02
Rockville, MD 20875
301-443-5158
www.nimh.nih.gov

Freedom from Fear
Avenue 308
Staten Island, NY 10305

National Mental Health Association
1021 Prince Street
Alexandria, VA 22314
800-969-NMHA
www.nmha.org

Agoraphobics in Motion (AIM)
1719 Crooks
Royal Oak, MI 48067-1306
1-248-547-0400

Agoraphobics Building Independent Lives, Inc (ABIL)
3805 Cutshaw Avenue, Suite 415
Richmond, VA 23230 1-804-353-3964

Next
Depression is covered in the next chapter.

References and Reading List:

American Psychiatric Association. *Diagnostic and statistical manual of mental disorders.* Fourth edition. Washington, D.C.: American Psychiatric Press, 1994.

Beidel, D.C., and Horak, F.B. "Behavior therapy for vestibular rehabilitation." *Journal of Anxiety Disorders,* 15:121-130, 2001.

Cass, S.P., and Furman, J.M. *Balance disorders: A case-study approach.* Philadelphia: F.A. Davis Company, 1996.

Clark, M.R., and Swartz, K.L. "A conceptual structure and methodology for the systematic approach to the evaluation and treatment of patients with chronic dizziness." *Journal of Anxiety Disorders,* 15:95-106, 2001.

Hales, R.E., Yudofsky, S.C., and Talbott, J.A. *The American psychiatric press textbook of psychiatry,* Third edition. Washington, D.C.: American Psychiatric Press, 1999.

Sklare, D.A., Konrad, H.R., Maser, J.D., and Jacob, R.G. "Special issue on the interface of balance disorders and anxiety: an introduction and overview." *Journal of Anxiety Disorders,* 15:1-7, 2001.

Staabe, J.P. "Diagnosis and treatment of psychologic symptoms and psychiatric disorders in patients with dizziness and imbalance." *Otolaryngologic Clinics of North America, 33(3):617-635, 2000.*

Townsend, M.C. *Psychiatric mental health nursing: Concepts of care.* Third edition. Philadelphia: F.A Davis Company, 2000.

Varcarolis, E.M. *Foundations of psychiatric mental health nursing: A clinical approach.* Fourth edition. Philadelphia: W.B. Saunders Company, 2002.

Yardley, L. "Overview of psychologic effects of chronic dizziness and balance disorders." *Otolaryngologic Clinics of North America,* 33(3):603-616, 2000.

Yardley, L., Britten, J., Lear, S., and Bird, J. "Relationship between balance system function and agoraphobic avoidance." *Behavior Research Therapy,* 33:435-439, 1995.

Yardley, L., Luxon, L., and Haake, N.P. "A longitudinal study of symptoms, anxiety, and subjective well-being in patients with vertigo." *Clinical Otolaryngology*, 19:109-116, 1994.

Chapter Forty-nine
Depression

Feeling blue or down, once in a while, is part of life. Being so blue it's no longer possible to find pleasure in usual activities or being a bit blue or down constantly, for two years or more are abnormal and may be diagnosed as depression.

If you have thoughts of hurting yourself or ending your life PUT THIS BOOK DOWN AND GET HELP. Call a suicide hotline, your PCP. Don't try to fight the hopelessness and despair on your own.

How Common?
Depression is fairly common and present in about 3-5% of Americans at any given point in time. Men have a 5-12% chance of developing depression sometime during their lives and women a 10-25% risk.

Depression is even more common in people with chronic diseases, including those with vestibular disorders. One Meniere's disease study found that 80% of those actively having attacks and 39% of those not currently having attacks were depressed.

The Symptoms
Some of the symptoms of depression in adults:

- Anger
- Anxiety
- Constipation/diarrhea
- Decreased libido
- Don't care how they look
- Fatigue
- Feeling helpless
- Feeling hopeless
- Feeling worthless
- Fidgeting
- Finger tapping
- Guilt

- Inactivity
- Irritability
- Lethargy
- Poor sleep
- Poor appetite
- Sleeping too much
- Slow movement
- Slow speech
- Slow to understand
- Smoking

Some of the symptoms depressed children may experience:

- Anger
- Boredom
- Constantly on the move
- Crankiness
- Crying for no reason
- Fighting
- Fidgeting
- Irritability
- Moodiness
- Restlessness
- Resting frequently
- Sad
- Talking excessively
- Tired or listless

What Causes Depression?

Many things can cause depression including biological factors, drugs, genetics, medical conditions, medications, nutritional deficiencies, and psychosocial events or problems (events and situations affecting thought and mood).

Biological theory

Depression is a disruption of the brain's neurotransmitters. This disruption can occur from genetics, drugs, bodily diseases or disorders of thought/mood. The neurotransmitters that may be affected include norepinephrine, dopamine, serotonin, acetylcholine and GABA.

Drugs

Several drugs have been implicated in depression including barbiturates (Phenobarbital), steroids (prednisone), antipsychotics, benzodiazepines (Valium, Xanax, Ativan), caffeine, propranolol (Inderal), cimetidine (Tagamet), alcohol and some anti-cancer drugs.

Genetics

A tendency toward depression seems to run in some families. In some cases even twins raised apart in different homes with different families have been found to share depression, pointing to a physical cause rather than living conditions.

Medical conditions

A number of medical conditions can cause depression including migraine, multiple sclerosis, hydrocephalus, Addison s disease, Cushing s disease, stroke, hypothyroidism, hypoparathyroidism, hyperparathyroidism, flu, hepatitis, mononucleosis, pneumonia, rheumatoid arthritis, Sjögren s syndrome, systemic lupus erythamotosus, anemia, and electrolyte imbalance, particularly increased or decreased potassium.

Nutritional deficiency

Diets deficient in certain nutrients may also cause depression. These deficiencies include lack of vitamin B1, vitamin B12, niacin, zinc, folic acid, vitamin C and/or protein.

Psychosocial theories

- Psychoanalytical theory: Internally directed rage due to the loss of something
- Learning theory: Learned helplessness
- Object loss theory: Abandoned before 6 months of age
- Cognitive theory: Problem with thought that leads to a defeated attitude.
- Transactional model theory: This theory sees depression as the result of a combination of causes.

Treatment

Depression is very real and can have a very powerful grip on a person. Beating it can require professional help. This help can come from a PCP, psychiatrist, psychologist, psychiatric nurse practitioner, or psychiatric social worker.

There are a number of treatments available including diet change, medication change, treatment of medically caused depression, therapy/counseling, antidepression medications and a few alternative therapies. The treatment(s) used depends upon the cause of the depression and how the treating health care professional views depression and it's causes.

The drugs in common use include the tricyclic antidepressant drug family and selective serotonin uptake inhibitors.

The counseling/therapy approaches used most often include brief psychodynamic therapy, cognitive therapy, interpersonal therapy and/or cognitive-behavior therapy.

Some alternative depression treatments include St. John's Wart, exercise and transcranial stimulation.

Sum Up

Depression is a condition every bit as real as disorders of other body areas. It can totally disrupt a person's life, particularly when left untreated. Help is out there and should be sought out the same way diagnosis and treatment of other body areas are.

Next

Fatigue is covered in the next chapter.

References and Reading List:

Coker, N.J., Coker, R.R., Jenkins, H.A., and Vincent, K.R. "Psychological profile of patients with Meniere's disease." *Archives of Otolaryngology Head and Neck Surgery*, 115(11):1355-1357, 1989.

Soderman, A.H., Bagger-Sjoback, D., Bergenius, J., and Langius, A. "Factors influencing quality of life in patients with Meniere's Disease, identified by a multidimensional approach." *Otology and Neurotology*, 23:941-948, 2002.

Townsend, M.C. *Psychiatric mental health nursing: Concepts of Care.* Third edition. Philadelphia: F.A Davis Company, 2000.

Yardley, L. "Overview of psychologic effects of chronic dizziness and balance disorders." *Otolaryngologic Clinics of North America,* 33(3):603-616, 2000.

Chapter Fifty
Fatigue

Many people with vestibular disorders experience fatigue, that "too tired to do much of anything" sort of feeling. Like most issues surrounding vestibular disorders, fatigue hasn't been studied in detail so little is known to a scientific certainty about why it occurs and who is most likely to experience it.

Fatigue, in some people, goes way beyond feeling tired, getting a good night's sleep and waking up good to go in the morning. It's waking up each morning feeling so tired it's hard to believe they've been to bed. Too tired to prepare elaborate meals, too tired to work, too tired to do school work, too tired to get through the day without a nap or many naps. Too tired to care about life in general.

Fatigue can also impair balance. Remember that good balance requires an alert mind. When fatigued the mind may no longer be alert enough to maintain a proper level of balance ability and that, in turn, may lead to even more fatigue setting up a vicious cycle.

Fatigue can be a huge factor in the life of someone with a vestibular disorder. It can affect both quality of life and balance function.

Theories

Fatigue has many explanations, and one person can have more than one cause for their fatigue.

The general strain of feeling unwell while trying to carry on a modern life can cause fatigue.

Anxiety can produce fatigue. Not only can a person become anxious when they think about their vestibular disorder and it's symptoms but bad vestibular signals can directly stimulate the autonomic nervous system resulting directly in anxiety. Being all revved up and ready to flee or fight it out can sap a person's energy very quickly.

The lack of proper sleep can lead rapidly to fatigue in anyone. Poor sleep in someone with a vestibular disorder can increase symptoms and decrease balance ability. Vertigo and other vestibular symptoms themselves can occur while in bed, disturbing sleep and causing fatigue.

Fatigue is very commonly seen in depression and depression is common in people with chronic medical conditions, including vestibular disorders.

The dehydration and an electrolyte imbalance that occur from the vomiting, sweating and diarrhea accompanying violent attacks of vertigo or as a side effect when water pills are used in Meniere's disease and other forms of endolymphatic hydrops can lead to fatigue.

A poor or inadequate diet can cause fatigue because the body isn't getting the fuel it needs to carry out its normal business. Nausea, vomiting and/or poor appetite can all interfere with proper nutrition.

Both sleepiness and fatigue are common when first taking vestibular suppressants and may go on for extended periods of time in some people. This can get to the point of interfering with both thought and the activities of daily living.

One time loss of vestibular function causes the brain to struggle quite a bit as it reorganizes the way it both uses vestibular information and carries out balance. This struggle causes fatigue. Once the reorganization is complete the fatigue may go away or at least improve.

Fatigue can cause even more fatigue by undoing chemical compensation, the brain's way of reorganizing after a partial vestibular loss of function.

Fatigue may also occur directly from a vestibular disorder. If the vestibular disorder causes constantly fluctuating levels of balance function fatigue may be constant too. When balance function changes profoundly for a short period of time, like during a violent attack of Meniere's disease, it's not uncommon for a person to sleep for hours on end due to profound fatigue.

Combating Fatigue

Before making any large lifestyle changes to deal with the fatigue, discuss it with a PCP. Give a doctor the opportunity to look for other causes of fatigue that might require different treatment.

In general, fatigue management includes:

- A well-balanced diet spread out over the day and beginning with breakfast
- Drinking enough water over the course of the day
- Adequate amounts of nightly sleep
- Stress management
- Daily exercise
- Good time management with work spread out over the day with time for rest. Don't bite off more than you can chew each day.
- Rest up well before a big event and schedule rest breaks, even if it means sitting in a parked car or in the bathroom for a short while.
- A nap can help at times

Reduce or manage stress when possible. Exercise is one stress management tool that can reduce fatigue in some people. Take as few vestibular suppressants as possible and DO NOT drink alcohol during a day a suppressant has been taken. When depression is present, counseling and possibly drug therapy can be helpful.

Sum Up

Fatigue can be caused by vestibular disorders and lead to an increase in vestibular symptoms and reduced balance ability. Steps can be taken that may lessen or stop the fatigue in some people. As long as vestibular function is fluctuating and producing symptoms fatigue will most likely be around.

Next

Stress is covered in the next chapter.

References and Reading List:

Cohen, H., Ewell, L.R., and Jenkins, H.A. "Disability in Meniere's Disease." *Archives of Otolaryngology-Head and Neck Surgery*, 121:29-33, 1995.

Schlesinger, A., Redfern, M.S., Dahl, R.E., and Jennings, J.R. "Postural control, attention and sleep deprivation." *Neuroreport*, 9(1):49-52, 1998.

Chapter Fifty-one
Stress

Stress is any event or situation that interferes with the normal physical and/or mental or emotional function of the body. It's being confronted with more than you can physically or mentally handle. Vestibular disorders and their effects are certainly stressful. In addition disease, injury, symptoms of disease or injury, drugs, difficult relationships, peer pressure, school, competition, driving, hot weather and cold weather can also cause stress.

Effect on the Body
The immediate effect of stress is the release of the catecholamine chemicals, including adrenaline (chemical name: epinephrine), throughout the body. This chemical release quickly prepares a person for a fight or flight response by increasing heart rate, blood pressure, alertness, and releasing glucose into the blood stream.

When stress continues for long periods of time, steroids in larger than normal amounts, enter the blood stream causing salt and water retention, increased blood sugar levels, breakdown of body protein and fat, increased fatty acid levels in the blood stream, increased blood pressure and increases in blood volume. These changes are hard on the body. When allowed to go on for long periods of time they can lead to blood clots, heart disease, brain attack (newer term for stroke), high blood pressure and may even interfere with the body's immune system.

The Inner Ear Effect
There are a number of ways that stress may effect inner ear function or cause symptoms.

Body wide retention of salt and water may cause an increased amount of endolymph in the inner ear of people with endolymphatic hydrops (including Meniere's disease) leading to an increase in the number of symptoms and/or their intensity.

Sodium and water retention can also lead to an increase in the fluid pressure around the brain. This increased pressure can cause symptoms by disturbing already damaged areas of the inner ear. It can also cause an abnormal opening between the inner ear and the middle ear called a perilymph fistula.

The symptoms of brain problems such as hydrocephalus, pseudotumor cerebri and Arnold-Chiari type I can also be increased by salt and water retention.

Elevated blood sugar levels can lead to increases in inner ear fluids. If the blood sugar level fluctuates the symptoms can increase and decrease in severity also.

Thickening of the blood may interfere with inner ear circulation or blood flow to the vestibulocochlear nerve. A blood clot could also totally cut off circulation to these areas resulting in cell death.

The increase in fatty acid levels can lead to cholesterol deposits in blood vessels including those supplying the ear, the vestibulocochlear nerve and the brain. Blood flow to these areas could be slowed down or even stopped.

Excess amounts of steroids and adrenaline in the blood stream can lead to immune system problems. This could allow viruses to flourish in the inner ear or set off an autoimmune disorder. The possibility also exists that increased levels of steroids and/or adrenaline right in the inner ear may also lead to physical changes and symptoms.

Compensation, in people who already have a partial loss of vestibular function, can begin to unravel under stress. Vestibular compensation is the chemical process occurring in the brain that allows it to carry on after a partial vestibular loss.

Stress can also lead to behavior that in turn causes vestibular problems. Drinking alcohol, having too much caffeine (coffee, chocolate), eating too many refined carbohydrates (candy, cookies, bread, and pasta) and overeating on salt can cause vestibular symptoms in some people.

Last, a vestibular disorder itself can be stressful and may set up a never ending cycle of stress worsening the vestibular disorder which in turn increases the stress level.

Coping With Stress

A person can try to ignore stress, attempt to remove it from their life, do things that reduce the stress or it's effects, use stress to their advantage (when possible), rethink how they look at stressful situations and events, seek treatment for the problems and symptoms stress has created, and/or undergo counseling or therapy to improve their situation.

Day to day stress is a part of the human condition. Removing all of it and still being a part of the world isn't a reasonable possibility. The issue isn't so much if we have stress, but how we handle, treat or use the stress we have.

Simply ignoring stress works for some people but for others this approach spells trouble. The long-term effects of stress can be just too serious to ignore.

Removing all stress sounds good in theory but in reality a person would just about have to leave the world, as they knew it and crawl into a cave to be free of the stresses of modern life.

Another approach to stress is focusing on the problems it has created and not it's cause. This method is in pretty widespread use not because it's the best but because it's just easier to forget about looking for the stressors in life and focus only on the ugly problems and symptoms it has created.

Some stress comes from within a person and is the result of how they actually feel about various things. In every situation figure out what can be changed, what can't be and what's worth the fight. Is the thing that's stressing you out really important? Is it worth getting all worked up over? How does it compare to severe world conditions like war, hunger, or famine?

For example, instead of getting annoyed on the highway by slow drivers perhaps one could contemplate how much easier life is with a car and how it beats walking 10 or 20 miles. Or, if getting somewhere on time is crucial why not leave earlier? These and other approaches can be explored alone or through counseling or therapy.

The effects of stress can be limited by a number of approaches including just plain getting out and having some fun, a good program of exercise for about 30 minutes three times each week, yoga, relaxation therapy, listening to music, setting aside time to just plain relax, getting enough sleep, guided imagery, hobbies and talking about stressful situations with people who understand what you're talking about. In some situations drug therapy may also be suggested and is safest when an experienced therapist (with the authority to write prescriptions) is directing the care and writing the prescriptions.

Problem Area
Not every health care professional views vestibular disorders or stress as physical problems. Some may, in fact, think it's all in a person's mind or some sort of personality weakness or character flaw. If stress seems to be associated with the vestibular disorder it might be viewed as a mental rather than as a physical problem. In this situation getting appropriate treatment can be difficult and may require looking for a different doctor or health care provider.

Sum Up
Stress is a part of the human condition and for many people is also a part of vestibular disorders. Some steps can be taken to reduce its impact.

Next
Thought and memory are covered in the next chapter.

References and Reading List

Andersson, G., and Yardley, L. "Time-series analysis of the relationship between dizziness and stress." *Scandanavian Journal of Psychology,* 41(1):49-54, 2000.

Marieb, E.N. *Human Anatomy and Physiology.* Fifth edition. San Francisco, California: Benjamin Cummings, 2000.

Rice, V.H. *Handbook of Stress, Coping and Health: Implications for nursing research, theory and practice.* Walnut Creek, California:Altamira Press, 2000.

Townsend, M.C. *Psychiatric Mental Health Nursing: Concepts of Care.* Third edition. Philadelphia: F.A Davis Company, 2000.

Yardley, L., Watson, S., Britton, J., Lear, S., and Bird, J. "Effects of anxiety arousal and mental stress on the vestibulo-ocular reflex." *Acta Otolaryngologica,* 15:597-602, 1995.

Chapter Fifty-two
Thought and Memory

Some people with severe or chronic vestibular disorders talk about having "no memory" or that they "can't think straight." This, in addition to feelings of unreality and fatigue, is sometimes referred to by people with vestibular disorders as "brain fog."

These symptoms are a problem for obvious reasons and for one not so visible, most doctors and health care professionals outside the vestibular specialty are not aware this goes on and may not link it to a vestibular disorder.

Unfortunately there's been very little research on the topic. In one of the few studies on the issue Yardley found poor concentration in 21% of people with mild dizziness and in 10% of people who were "normal." Dr. Yardley's conclusion was that this "may reflect the need for dizzy patients to expend extra mental effort on the perception of orientation and control of movement."

Theories

There may not be much scientific information available about this problem but there are many theories. Fatigue, stress, depression, drugs, and as Dr. Yardley stated, vestibular disorders themselves have all been implicated as the cause.

The fatigue of a vestibular disorder alone can lead to difficulty with both thought and memory. It can also cause an increase in symptoms leading to more fatigue and difficulty thinking and remembering things.

Stress and anxiety from any cause can lead to trouble with decision-making, thought and memory. It may also lead to a worsening of the disorder that in turn can lead to an increase in problems with thought and memory.

People with chronic diseases, including vestibular disorders, frequently become depressed. Depression has long been known to cause thought and memory problems.

Many of the drugs used to suppress vestibular symptoms do their work in the brain and are classified as central nervous system depressants. They reduce the brain's ability to think in an organized manner and to remember things, events, people, etc.

A diuretic can also be a problem if it causes dehydration and/or an electrolyte imbalance. Both can cause trouble thinking or remembering things and if severe enough can even lead to confusion.

Vertigo can be a very strong, nasty sensation capable of taking the full attention of a person, letting them think of little else.

Thought and memory problems can also come directly from a vestibular disorder. These disorders don't cause brain damage but may force the brain to use more space or energy for balance and figuring out position in space and less for thought and memory.

How bad this will be, and how long it will last, depends upon the disorder and if it's partial, complete or fluctuating. In the case of a partial loss the thought and memory problems should be temporary. In a large, two-sided loss, it may be long lasting. Disorders with fluctuations taking place weeks or months apart allow people to get back to something close to normal in-between. Unfortunately if the fluctuations are occurring just hours or days apart the thought and memory problems may be constant or nearly so.

What Can Be Done?

Of course removing the cause of the thought and memory problem would be best, but isn't always possible. When it can't be done some changes might be beneficial.

Drugs

All drug related issues should be discussed fully with the prescribing doctor or primary care provider. Through trial and error a drug with fewer problems may be found. For example if fatigue is a problem a switch from Dramamine Original Formula to Dramamine Less Drowsy might be helpful.

Be very careful about using alcohol when taking drugs. Don't drink any alcohol when taking a central nervous system depressant drug such as Dramamine, meclizine, or Valium. Always read the instructions that come with a drug.

Diuretics

Drink plenty of fluids when taking a diuretic. Drink even more water if losing body fluids from a long period of vomiting or diarrhea, when suffering through a cold or the flu or when working or exercising outdoors in heat or humidity. A person should not deprive themselves of food or fluids when taking diuretics.

Balance/Brain

To help the brain during compensation, the period of brain reorganization, be as generally fit as possible. Do activities that develop and keep strong muscles and flexible joints. Under the supervision of a doctor and/or physical therapist find exercises and activities that improve vestibular function, vision and proprioception. Make sure vision is checked yearly and glasses worn as instructed.

Coping

Sometimes the only steps that can be taken to deal with thought, memory problems and "brain fog" are lifestyle changes.

Some general suggestions:

- Thought and memory problems can be made worse by lack of sleep, fatigue, drugs and alcohol. Getting enough sleep and avoiding drugs that aggravate it will be helpful.
- Have paper and pencil ready to make reminder notes. Refer to these notes at set times, be organized and compulsive about it.
- Don't live in a dark, sound proofed room, away from contact with other people but do decrease noise, change your lighting, invite less people to social events to lessen the fog and its impact.

- Don't make big decisions when tired
- Rest up well before a big or important event
- Take breaks during a big event—get away from the sound and visual excitement. Even sitting down in a restroom or parked car for a while can help
- If you are too brain fogged to work, you're probably too brain fogged to drive a car
- Memorization and other learning should be done in small doses. Study for several minutes at a time many times throughout the day for days to weeks to learn something.
- If decision-making is difficult learn a systematic way to go about it. This can be learned from books and courses or passed along through mentoring. In addition to helping during an illness this skill can help in other aspects of life.
- Be in the easiest environment where you are at your best when doing important thinking. Sitting in a comfortable chair with your head supported, or even laying down helps some people.
  Students: Don't even think about cramming or pulling an all-nighter for a test—study in advance and and get a full nights sleep before a test.

Sum Up

Both thought and memory can be affected in a person under treatment for a vestibular disorder. Treatment and coping depend on the cause in each individual case.

References and Reading List:

Andersson, G., Hagman, J., Talianzadeh, R., Svedberg, A., and Larsen, H.C. "Dual-task study of cognitive and postural interference in patients with vestibular disorders." *Otology and Neurotology*, 24(2):289-93, 2003.

Andersson, G., Hagnebo, C., and Yardley, L. "Stress and symptoms of Meniere's disease: a time series analysis." *Journal of Psychosomatic Research*, 43:595-603, 1997.

Andersson, G., Yardley, L., and Luxon, L. "A dual task study of interference between mental activity and control of balance." *American Journal of Otology*, 19:632-637, 1998.

Yardley, L., Burgneay, J., Nazareth, I., and Luxon, L. "Neuro-otological and psychiatric abnormalities in a community sample of people with dizziness: a blind, controlled investigation." *Journal of Neurology, Neurosurgery and Psychiatry*, 65(5):679-84, 1998.

Yardley, L., Gardner, M., Bronstein, A., Davies, R., Buckwell, D., and Luxon, L. "Interference between postural control and mental task performance in patients with vestibular disorder and healthy controls." *Journal of Neurology, Neurosurgery, and Psychiatry*, 71:48-52, 2001.

Yardley, L., Papo, D., Bronstein, A., Gresty, M., Gardner, M., Lavie, N., and Luxon, L. "Attentional demands of continuously monitoring orientation using vestibular information." *Neuropsychologia*, 40(4):373-383, 2002.

In Conclusion

Many vestibular disorders exist and they can be difficult to diagnose, treat and get rid of. There are many treatments and doctors but it can take a bit of time and hard work to find the right ones.

Getting more information

First and foremost use your health providers as your primary source of information. If you need more read this and the other books available on the topic.

Visit a medical school library to find more advanced books on the topic. Two excellent libraries in the U.S. are the Leroy A. Schall Library of Otolaryngology at the Massachusetts Eye and Ear Infirmary in Boston MA, www.meei.harvard.edu/info/library.php and the Athalie Irvine Clarke library at the House Ear Institute in Los Angeles, CA. In the U.K. the RNID owns a library run by the University College London (UCL) and located at the Institute of Laryngology and Otology, a department of UCL in the Royal National Throat, Nose and Ear Hospital, 330-332 Gray's Inn Road, London WCIX 8EE, Telephone: 020 7915 1553, Textphone: 020 7915 1553, Fax: 020 7915 1443, www.rnid.org.uk

There are many reputable sources of information on the Internet but buyer beware, there are many sources of bogus information as well. Some good places to start on the Internet are the Vestibular Disorders Association at www.vestibular.org, The National Institute on Deafness and Other Communicative Disorders (NIDCD) at www.nicdc.nih.gov and the authors webpage at www.balance-and-dizziness.com

Medical and scientific journal articles can be located using the National Library of Medicine's PubMed at www.ncbi.nlm.nih.gov/entrez/query.fcgi?DB=pubmed. The web page includes a tutorial and information about it's use.

INDEX

vestibulopathy, 165
vision, 16, 17, 18, 65, 174, 184
von Hippel-Lindau Disease, 167
VOR, 16, 17, 18, 34, 36, 37, 41, 65
VORTEQ, 37
VRT, 63, 64, 65, 66, 72
whiplash, 95
word recognition test, 38

Made in the USA
Lexington, KY
17 February 2010